Medical Medium B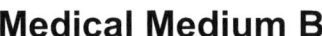

Con Mich

Neurology

neurology, scientific distinctiveness involved with the frightened device and its useful or natural issues. Neurologists diagnose and deal with illnesses and issues of the mind, spinal cord, and nerves.

The first medical research of nerve feature in animals had been executed within the early 18th century with the aid of using English physiologist Stephen Hales and Scottish physiologist Robert Whytt. Knowledge become won within the past due nineteenth century approximately the reasons of aphasia, epilepsy, and motor issues bobbing up from mind harm. French neurologist Jean-Martin Charcot and English neurologist William Gowers defined and categorized many illnesses of the frightened device. The mapping of the useful regions of the mind via selective electric stimulation additionally started out within the nineteenth century. Despite those contributions, however, maximum know-how of the mind and frightened capabilities got here from research in animals and from the microscopic evaluation of nerve cells.

The electroencephalograph (EEG), which data electric mind interest, become invented within the Twenties with the aid of using Hans Berger. Development of the EEG, evaluation of cerebrospinal fluid acquired with the aid of using lumbar puncture (spinal tap), and improvement of cerebral angiography allowed neurologists to growth the precision in their diagnoses and increase precise treatments and rehabilitative measures. Further helping the analysis and remedy of mind issues had been the improvement of automated axial tomography (CT) scanning within the early Nineteen Seventies and magnetic resonance imaging (MRI) within the 1980s, each of which yielded detailed, noninvasive perspectives of the internal of the mind. The identity of chemical dealers within the crucial frightened device and the elucidation in their roles in transmitting and blocking off nerve impulses have brought about the creation of a big range of medicinal drugs which could accurate or alleviate diverse neurological issues together with Parkinson disorder, a couple of sclerosis, and epilepsy. Neurosurgery, a scientific distinctiveness associated with neurology, has additionally benefited from CT scanning and different an increasing number of particular techniques of finding lesions and different abnormalities in frightened tissues.

Behavioral Neurology and Dementia

Alzheimer Disease

Practice Essentials

Alzheimer disorder (AD) is a neurodegenerative ailment marked with the aid of using cognitive and behavioral impairment that notably interferes with social and occupational functioning. It is an incurable disorder with an extended preclinical duration and revolutionary course. In AD, plaques increase within the hippocampus, a shape deep within the mind that allows to encode memories, and in different regions of the cerebral cortex which can be worried in wondering and making decisions. Whether plaques themselves reason AD or whether or not they're a derivative of the AD procedure stays unknown. The following picture depicts one of the cardinal neuroimaging findings in AD – hippocampal atrophy.

Signs and symptoms

Preclinical Alzheimer disorder

An affected person with preclinical AD can also additionally seem absolutely ordinary on bodily exam and intellectual popularity testing. Specific areas of the mind (e.g., entorhinal cortex, hippocampus) are probable to be affected a long time earlier than any symptoms and symptoms or signs and symptoms seem.

Mild Alzheimer disorder

Signs of slight AD can consist of the subsequent:

- Memory loss
- Confusion approximately the place of acquainted locations
- Taking longer to perform ordinary, everyday tasks
- Trouble managing cash and paying bills
- Compromised judgment, regularly main to awful decisions

- Loss of spontaneity and feel of initiative
- Mood and persona adjustments; extended anxiety

Moderate Alzheimer disorder

The signs and symptoms of this level can consist of the subsequent:

- Increasing reminiscence loss and confusion
- Shortened interest span
- Problems spotting pals and own circle of relative's members
- Difficulty with language; issues with reading, writing, running with numbers
- Difficulty organizing mind and wondering logically
- Inability to analyze new matters or to address new or sudden situations
- Restlessness, agitation, anxiety, tearfulness, wandering, specially within the past due afternoon or at night
- Repetitive statements or movement; occasional muscle twitches

- Hallucinations, delusions, suspiciousness or paranoia, irritability
- Loss of impulse manage: Shown via conduct including undressing at beside the point instances or locations or vulgar language
- Perceptual-motor issues: Such as problem getting out of a chair or putting the table

Severe Alzheimer disorder

Patients with intense AD can't understand own circle of relatives or cherished ones and can't speak effectively. They are absolutely depending on others for care, and all feel of self appears to vanish.

Other signs and symptoms of intense AD can consist of the subsequent:

- Weight loss
- Seizures, pores and skin infections, issue swallowing
- Groaning, moaning, or grunting

- Increased sleeping
- Lack of bladder and bowel manage

In give up-level AD, sufferers can be in mattress a lot or all the time. Death is regularly the end result of different illnesses, regularly aspiration pneumonia.

Diagnosis

Means of diagnosing AD consist of the subsequent:

- **Clinical exam:** The medical analysis of AD is commonly made all through the slight level of the disorder, the use of the above-indexed symptoms and symptoms
- **Lumbar puncture:** ranges of tau and phosphorylated tau within the cerebrospinal fluid are regularly expanded in AD, while amyloid ranges are commonly low; at gift, however, habitual size of CSF tau and amyloid isn't always advocated besides in studies settings
- **Imaging research:** Imaging research are specially crucial for ruling out probably

treatable reasons of revolutionary cognitive decline, including persistent subdural hematoma or ordinary-strain hydrocephalus. Moreover, volumetric research of the hippocampus and 2-[18F] fluoro-2-Deoxy-D-glucose positron emission tomography (FDG-PET) without or with amyloid imaging were hired for early detection and differentiating dementia etiologies.

Management

All pills authorized with the aid of using America Food and Drug Administration (FDA) for the remedy of AD are symptomatic treatments that modulate neurotransmitters, both acetylcholine or glutamate. The popular scientific remedy for AD consists of cholinesterase inhibitors (ChEIs) and a partial N-Methyl-D-aspartate (NMDA) antagonist. They do now no longer deal with the underlying reason of AD nor halt the charge of decline.

The following instructions of psychotropic medicinal drugs were used to deal with the secondary signs and symptoms of AD, including despair, agitation, aggression, hallucinations, delusions, and sleep issues:

- Antidepressants
- Anxiolytics
- Antiparkinsonian dealers
- Beta-blockers
- Antiepileptic pills
- Neuroleptics
- Amyloid-directed antibody

Prevention

There aren't any established modalities for stopping AD, however proof, in large part epidemiologic, shows that wholesome life can lessen the hazard of growing the disorder; the subsequent can be protecting:

- Physical interest
- Exercise
- Cardiorespiratory fitness

Diet: Although no definitive nutritional pointers may be made, in general, dietary styles that seem useful for AD prevention match the Mediterranean diet

Background

Alzheimer disorder (AD) is the maximum not unusual place shape of dementia. In the US alone, about 6.08 million Americans had both medical AD or slight cognitive impairment because of AD in 2017. That range is predicted to develop to fifteen million with the aid of using 2060. AD is the 6th main reason of loss of life within the United States, accounting for three.6% of all deaths in 2014. The percent of Alzheimer's decedents who died in a scientific facility (e.g., hospital) declined from 14.7% in 1999 to 6.6% in 2014, while the proportion who died at domestic extended from 13.9% in 1999 to 24.9% in 2014. Economically, AD is a primary public fitness problem. Total bills in 2017 for fitness care and lengthy-time period take care of all people with AD or different dementias are anticipated at $259 billion. By 2050, those charges should upward push as excessive as $1.1 trillion.

Currently, a post-mortem or mind biopsy is the handiest manner to make a definitive analysis of AD. In medical practice, the analysis is commonly made on the premise of the records and findings on Mental Status Examination.

Symptomatic treatments are the handiest remedies to be had for AD. The popular scientific remedies consist of cholinesterase inhibitors and a partial N -Methyl-D-aspartate (NMDA) antagonist. Psychotropic medicinal drugs are regularly used to deal with secondary signs and symptoms of AD, including despair, agitation, and sleep issues.

Historical background

In 1901, a German psychiatrist named Alois Alzheimer determined an affected person on the Frankfurt Asylum named Mrs. Auguste D. This 51-12 months-antique lady suffered from a lack of short-time period reminiscence, amongst different behavioral signs and symptoms that confused Dr. Alzheimer. Five years later, in April 1906, the affected person died, and Dr. Alzheimer dispatched her mind and her scientific data to Munich, in which he become running within the lab of Dr. Emil Kraeplin. By staining sections of her mind within the laboratory, he become capable of pick out amyloid plaques and neurofibrillary tangles.

A speech given with the aid of using Dr. Alzheimer on November three, 1906, become the primary time the pathology and the medical signs and symptoms of the ailment, which on the time become termed presenile dementia, had been supplied collectively. Alzheimer posted his findings in 1907.

In the beyond 15-two decades, dramatic development has been made in expertise the neurogenetics and pathophysiology of AD. Four exclusive genes were definitively related to AD, and others which have a possible function were diagnosed. The mechanisms with the aid of using which altered amyloid and tau protein metabolism, irritation, oxidative strain, and hormonal adjustments can also additionally produce neuronal degeneration in AD are being elucidated, and rational pharmacologic interventions primarily based totally on those discoveries are being advanced.

Anatomy

Healthy neurons have an inner help shape in part made from systems referred to as microtubules. These microtubules act like tracks, guiding vitamins and molecules from the frame of the cellular right all the way down to the ends of the axon and back. A unique form of protein, tau, binds to the microtubules and stabilizes them.

In AD, tau is modified chemically. It starts offevolved to pair with different threads of tau, which come to be tangled collectively. When this happens, the microtubules disintegrate, collapsing the neuron's shipping device (see the picture below). The formation of those neurofibrillary tangles (NFTs) can also additionally end result first in malfunctions in verbal exchange among neurons and later within the loss of life of the cells.

In addition to NFTs, the anatomic pathology of AD consists of senile plaques (SPs; additionally, called beta-amyloid plaques) on the microscopic degree and cerebrocortical atrophy on the macroscopic degree (see the picture below). The hippocampus and medial temporal lobe are the preliminary web sites of tangle deposition and atrophy. This may be visible on mind magnetic resonance imaging early in AD and allows help a medical analysis.

SPs and NFTs had been defined with the aid of using Alois Alzheimer in his authentic document at the ailment in 1907. They are actually universally regularly occurring because the pathological hallmark of the disorder.

Pathophysiology

A continuum exists among the pathophysiology of ordinary growing old and that of AD. Pathologic hallmarks of AD were diagnosed; however, those capabilities additionally arise within the brains of cognitively intact folks. For example, in an observe wherein neuropathologists had been blinded to medical facts, they diagnosed 76% of brains of cognitively intact aged sufferers as demonstrating AD.

AD influences the three methods that preserve neurons wholesome: verbal exchange, metabolism, and repair. Certain nerve cells within the mind prevents running, lose connections with different nerve cells, and sooner or later die. The destruction and loss of life of those nerve cells reasons the reminiscence failure, persona adjustments, issues in wearing out every day activities, and different capabilities of the disorder.

The accumulation of SPs frequently precedes the medical onset of AD. NFTs, lack of neurons, and lack of synapses accompany the development of cognitive decline.

Considerable interest has been dedicated to elucidating the composition of SPs and NFTs to discover clues approximately the molecular pathogenesis and biochemistry of AD. The foremost constituent of NFTs is the microtubule-related protein tau. In AD, hyperphosphorylated tau accumulates within the perikarya of massive and medium pyramidal neurons. Somewhat surprisingly, mutations of the tau gene end result now no longer in AD however in a few familial instances of frontotemporal dementia.

Since the time of Alois Alzheimer, SPs were recognized to consist of a starchlike (or amyloid) substance, commonly within the middle of those lesions. The amyloid substance is surrounded with the aid of using a halo or layer of degenerating (dystrophic) neurites and reactive glia (each astrocytes and microglia).

One of the maximum crucial advances in current a long time has been the chemical characterization of this amyloid protein, the sequencing of its amino acid chain, and the cloning of the gene encoding its precursor protein (on chromosome 21). These advances have supplied a wealth of records approximately the mechanisms underlying amyloid deposition within the mind, together with records approximately the familial varieties of AD.

Alzheimer disorder biomarkers can also additionally observe a sequential sample within the mind, consistent with a observe of AD biomarker trajectories. The observe blanketed each symptomatic and asymptomatic providers of autosomal dominant gene mutations connected to AD, together with APP, PSEN1, and PSEN2. Researchers did now no longer cope with tauopathy. Results display that amyloid deposition within the mind happens first, observed with the aid of using a decline in glucose metabolism after which structural mind atrophy. The charge of Ab accumulation become notably better in mutation providers as in comparison to noncarriers, and become located to start greater than 2 a long time earlier than the predicted onset of dementia. In providers, metabolism started out to lower at an average of 14.1 years earlier than predicted symptom onset, and structural adjustments within the mind started out 4.7 years earlier than predicted symptom onset. It is crucial to be aware that handiest approximately 1% of sufferers with AD have an autosomal dominant mutation, so consequences might not be generalizable to sporadic AD.

Although the amyloid cascade speculation has collected the maximum studies financing, different thrilling hypotheses were proposed. Among those are the mitochondrial cascade speculation.

In addition to NFTs and SPs, many different lesions of AD were identified due to the fact that Alzheimer's authentic papers had been posted. These consist of the granulovacuolar degeneration of Shimkowicz; the neuropil threads of Braak et al; and neuronal loss and synaptic degeneration, which can be concept to in the end mediate the cognitive and behavioral manifestations of the ailment.

In 2019, researchers diagnosed a brand new form of dementia that mimics AD however this is as a result of some other mechanism within the mind. This new category is limbic-important age-associated TDP-forty-three encephalopathy, (LATE). TDP-forty-three is a protein that allows adjust gene expression within the mind and different tissues, and while it misfolds it reasons issues within the mind. According to researchers, misfolded TDP-forty-three protein could be very not unusual place in older adults; approximately 25% of human's elderly eighty-five and older have sufficient misfolded TDP-forty three protein to have an effect on their reminiscence and wondering skills.

Neurofibrillary tangles and senile plaques

Plaques are dense, broadly speaking insoluble deposits of protein and mobile fabric out of doors and across the neurons. Plaques are manufactured from beta-amyloid (Ab), a protein fragment snipped from a bigger protein referred to as amyloid precursor protein (APP). These fragments clump collectively and are blended with different molecules, neurons, and non-nerve cells.

In AD, plaques increase within the hippocampus, a shape deep within the mind that allows to encode memories, and in different regions of the cerebral cortex which can be utilized in wondering and making decisions. Plaques can also additionally start to increase as early because the 5th decade of existence. Whether Ab plaques themselves reason AD or whether or not they're a derivative of the AD procedure continues to be unknown. It is thought that adjustments in APP shape can reason a rare, inherited shape of AD.

Tangles are insoluble twisted fibers that increase in the nerve cellular. Although many older humans increase a few plaques and tangles, the brains of humans with AD have them to a more quantity, especially in sure areas of the mind which can be crucial in reminiscence. There are probable to be huge age-associated variations withinthe quantity to which the presence of plaques and tangles are indicative of the presence of dementia.

NFTs are first of all and maximum densely disbursed within the medial component and within the pole of the temporal lobe; they have an effect on the entorhinal cortex and the hippocampus maximum severely (however, Braak et al located that during sporadic AD, tauopathy can also additionally seem first within the decrease brainstem in preference to within the transentorhinal place). As AD progresses, NFTs collect in lots of different cortical areas, starting in excessive-order affiliation areas and much less regularly within the number one motor and sensory areas.

SPs additionally collect frequently in affiliation cortices and within the hippocampus. Plaques and tangles have extraordinarily discrete and stereotypical styles of laminar distribution within the cerebral cortex, which suggest important involvement of corticocortical connections.

Although NFTs and SPs are function of AD, they're now no longer pathognomonic. NFTs are located in numerous different neurodegenerative issues, together with revolutionary supranuclear palsy and dementia pugilistica (persistent annoying encephalopathy). SPs can also additionally arise in ordinary growing old.

Therefore, the mere presence of those lesions isn't always enough to help the analysis of AD. These lesions ought to be found in enough numbers and in a function topographic distribution to satisfy the modern histopathologic standards for AD. There is consensus that the presence of even low numbers of NFTs within the cerebral neocortex with concomitant SPs is function of AD.

Some government believed that NFTs, while found in low densities and basically restricted to the hippocampus, had been a part of ordinary growing old. However, the histologic tiers for AD that Braak et al formulated consist of an early level wherein NFTs are gift at a low density within the entorhinal and perirhinal (i.e., transentorhinal) cortices. Therefore, even small numbers of NFTs in those regions of the medial temporal lobe can be bizarre.

Amyloid speculation as opposed to tau speculation

A crucial however arguable trouble within the pathogenesis of AD is the connection among amyloid deposition and NFT formation. Evidence indicates that bizarre amyloid metabolism performs a key pathogenic function. At excessive concentrations, the fibrillar shape of Ab has been proven to be neurotoxic to cultured neurons.

Cultured cortical and hippocampal neurons handled with Ab protein showcase adjustments function of apoptosis (self-regulated cellular destruction), together with nuclear chromatin condensation, plasma membrane blebbing, and internucleosomal DNA fragmentation. The fibrillar shape of Ab has additionally been proven to adjust the phosphorylation kingdom of tau protein.

The identity of numerous factor mutations within the APP gene in a few sufferers with early-onset familial AD and the improvement of transgenic mice displaying cognitive adjustments and SPs additionally incriminate Ab in AD. The apolipoprotein E (APOE) E4 allele, which has been connected with notably extended hazard for growing AD, can also additionally sell lack of ability to suppress manufacturing of amyloid, extended manufacturing of amyloid, or impaired clearance of amyloid with series out of doors of the neuron.

Autopsies have proven that sufferers with 1 or 2 copies of the APOE E4 allele generally tend to have greater amyloid. Additional proof comes from current experimental facts assisting the function of presenilins in Ab metabolism, in addition to findings of bizarre manufacturing of Ab protein in presenilin-mutation familial Alzheimer disorder.

Although very popular, the amyloid speculation isn't always uniformly regularly occurring. On autopsy evaluation, amyloid plaques can be undetectable within the brains of sufferers who had intense AD however can be gift within the brains of aged sufferers who did now no longer have dementia.

Dementia severity correlates higher with the range of neocortical NFTs than with SPs. The tau protein stabilizes neuronal microtubules. Destabilization of the microtubular device is purported to disrupt the Golgi apparatus, in flip inducing bizarre protein processing and growing manufacturing of Ab. In addition, this destabilization can also additionally lower axoplasmic flow, producing dystrophic neurites and contributing to synaptic loss.

Granulovacuolar degeneration and neuropil threads

Granulovacuolar degeneration happens nearly solely within the hippocampus. Neuropil threads are an array of dystrophic neurites diffusely disbursed within the cortical neuropil, greater or much less independently of plaques and tangles. This lesion shows neuropil changes past the ones simply because of NFTs and SPs and suggests a good greater vast insult to the cortical circuitry than that visualized with the aid of using reading handiest plaques and tangles.

Cholinergic neurotransmission and Alzheimer disorder

The cholinergic device is worried in reminiscence feature, and cholinergic deficiency has been implicated within the cognitive decline and behavioral adjustments of AD. Activity of the artificial enzyme choline acetyltransferase (CAT) and the catabolic enzyme acetylcholinesterase are notably decreased within the cerebral cortex, hippocampus, and amygdala in sufferers with AD.

The nucleus basalis of Meynert and diagonal band of Broca offer the principle cholinergic enter to the hippocampus, amygdala, and neocortex, which can be misplaced in sufferers with AD. Loss of cortical CAT and decline in acetylcholine synthesis in biopsy specimens were located to correlate with cognitive impairment and reaction-time performance. Because cholinergic disorder can also additionally make a contribution to the signs and symptoms of sufferers with AD, improving cholinergic neurotransmission constitutes a rational foundation for symptomatic remedy.

Oxidative strain and harm

Oxidative harm happens in AD. Studies have verified that a growth in oxidative harm selectively happens within the mind areas worried in regulating cognitive performance.

Oxidative harm probably serves as an early occasion that then initiates the improvement of cognitive disturbances and pathological capabilities determined in AD. A decline in protein synthesis competencies happens within the identical mind areas that showcase extended ranges of oxidative harm in sufferers with slight cognitive impairment (MCI) and AD. Protein synthesis can be one of the earliest mobile methods disrupted with the aid of using oxidative harm in AD.

Oxidative strain is thought to be a crucial issue in ordinary growing old and in neurodegenerative illnesses including Parkinson disorder, amyotrophic lateral sclerosis, and AD. Formation of unfastened carbonyls and thiobarbituric acid-reactive merchandise, an index of oxidative harm, are notably extended in AD mind tissue as in comparison with age-matched controls. Plaques and tangles show immunoreactivity to antioxidant enzymes.

Multiple mechanisms exist with the aid of using which mobile changes can be triggered with the aid of using oxidative strain, together with manufacturing of reactive oxygen species (ROS) within the cellular membrane (lipid peroxidation). This in flip impairs the diverse membrane proteins worried in ion homeostasis including N -Methyl-D-aspartate receptor channels or ion-reason adenosine triphosphatases.

The next growth in intracellular calcium, in conjunction with the buildup of ROS, damages diverse mobile additives including proteins, DNA, and lipids and might bring about apoptotic mobile loss of life.

Increased intracellular calcium can also adjust calcium-based enzyme interest including the implication of protein kinase C in amyloid protein metabolism and the phosphorylation of tau.

The involvement of calcium in AD has recommended that blocking off the growth in unfastened intracellular calcium can also additionally lessen neuronal harm. However, medical trials of nimodipine, a lipophilic calcium channel blocker this is mediated via inactivation of voltage-based L-kind (lengthy-lasting) calcium channels, have yielded normally disappointing consequences in sufferers with AD.

The apoptotic sample of mobile loss of life visible in oxidative strain is much like that produced with the aid of using Ab peptide publicity, and Ab neurotoxicity is attenuated with the aid of using antioxidants including nutrition E. Ab can also additionally result in toxicity with the aid of using enticing numerous binding web sites at the membrane floor. The receptor for superior glycation give up merchandise (RAGE) can be this sort of receptors. RAGE is a member of the immunoglobulin superfamily of cellular floor molecules recognized for its ability to bind superior glycation give up merchandise.

RAGE is likewise expressed in loads of different cellular types, together with endothelial cells and mononuclear phagocytes. Activation of this receptor is thought to cause mobile oxidative reactions. In addition, RAGE has been proven to mediate the interplay of Ab with glial cells, which can be one of the first steps within the inflammatory cascade.

Inflammatory reactions

Inflammatory and immune mechanisms can also additionally play a function within the degenerative procedure in AD. Reactive microglia are embedded in neuritic plaques. Increased cytokine ranges are visible within the serum, cortical plaques, and neurons of sufferers with AD, compared with elderly-matched manage sufferers. Interestingly, remodeling increase issue beta 1 (TGF-β1), that is an anti-inflammatory cytokine, has been located to sell or boost up the deposition of amyloid.

Classical supplement pathway fragments also are located within the brains of sufferers with AD, and amyloid can also additionally without delay set off the classical supplement pathway in an antibody-unbiased fashion.

Whether markers of immune and inflammatory methods actively take part within the neurodegenerative procedure or alternatively constitute an epiphenomenon stays unclear. Brain specimens from aged sufferers with arthritis handled with nonsteroidal anti-inflammatory pills (NSAIDs) have comparable numbers of senile plaques as do manage brains.

However, much less microglial activation is visible within the brains of the sufferers with arthritis. This shows that even though NSAIDs might not obstruct senile plaque formation, they will put off or save you medical signs and symptoms with the aid of using restricting the related irritation.

As referred to above, RAGE has been proven to mediate the interplay of amyloid and glial cells, generating mobile activation and an inflammatory reaction with cytokine manufacturing, chemotaxis, and haptotaxis. The expression of this receptor seems to be upregulated in neurons, vasculature, and microglia in affected areas of AD brains.

The unrelated elegance A scavenger receptor (elegance A SR) additionally mediates the adhesion of microglial cells to amyloid fibrils. SPs comprise excessive concentrations of microglia that specific elegance A SRs. RAGE and sophistication A SRs can also additionally constitute novel pharmacologic goals for diminishing the inflammatory and oxidative reactions related to AD.

Clusterin

Clusterin, a plasma protein, performs a crucial function within the pathogenesis of AD. In one observe, clusterin become related to atrophy of the entorhinal cortex, baseline disorder severity, and fast medical development in AD. This crucial observe shows that changes in amyloid chaperone proteins may be an applicable peripheral signature of AD. An observe with the aid of using Schrijvers et al notes that even though plasma clusterin ranges are notably related to baseline occurrence and severity of AD, they're now no longer associated with the hazard for AD.

Presenilins

A huge share of early-onset autosomal-dominant AD instances were connected to a candidate gene on chromosome 14 (14q24.3) referred to as presenilin-1 (PS1) and a candidate gene on chromosome 1 referred to as presenilin-2 (PS2). The 2 putative merchandise of those candidate genes, PS1 and PS2, proportion good sized amino-acid and structural similarities, suggesting that they will be functionally associated. In addition, the expression styles of PS1 and PS2 within the mind are comparable, if now no longer identical.

Both PS1 messenger RNA (mRNA) and PS2 mRNA are detectable handiest inside neuronal populations. Immunochemical analyses suggest that PS1 localizes to intracellular compartments, including the endoplasmic reticulum and the Golgi complex, which can be worried in comparable capabilities. Evidence helps the function of presenilins in Ab metabolism. Mice poor within the expression of PS1 showcase a dramatic lower in proteolytic cleavage of the transmembrane area of amyloid precursor protein (APP) with the aid of using secretase.

PS1 is immunoreactive with the neuritic issue of SPs. Both asymptomatic and demented topics wearing the PS1 mutation have extended manufacturing of the amyloidogenic Ab 42/43 isoform in pores and skin fibroblasts and plasma. Prominent deposition of Ab 42/43 is located in lots of mind areas of sufferers with PS1 mutations. These findings, in suggesting that inhibiting presenilin feature would possibly lower Ab amyloid manufacturing, provide new healing avenues.

Estrogen loss

Postmenopausal ladies are at better hazard than guys for AD. Some research has proven that estrogen loss can also additionally cause cognitive decline and neuronal degeneration, and the expression of nerve increase issue and mind-derived neurotrophic issue mRNA is likewise reduced.

Estrogen has additionally been proven to exert cytoprotective results and to save you amyloid toxicity in human neuroblastoma cellular cultures. However, a randomized medical trial of estrogen in cognitively ordinary ladies' elderly sixty-five years and older with a first-diploma relative with AD confirmed that estrogen remedy would possibly simply growth the hazard of stroke and dementia.

Etiology

The reason of AD is unknown. Several investigators now consider that converging environmental and genetic hazard elements cause a pathophysiologic cascade that, over a long time, results in Alzheimer pathology and dementia.

The following hazard elements for Alzheimer-kind dementia were diagnosed:

- Advancing age
- Family records
- APOE four genotype
- Obesity
- Insulin resistance
- Vascular elements
- Dyslipidemia
- Hypertension
- Inflammatory markers
- Down syndrome
- Traumatic mind harm

Midlife high blood pressure is a longtime hazard issue for past due-existence dementia, of which AD is the maximum not unusual place kind. A mind post-mortem observe comparing the hyperlink among high blood pressure and AD located that sufferers the use of beta-blockers to govern blood strain had fewer Alzheimer's-kind mind lesions on post-mortem as in comparison to sufferers taking no drug remedy or the ones taking different medicinal drugs.

In addition, epidemiologic research has recommended a few feasible hazard elements including aluminum and former despair. Other research has recommended protecting elements (e.g., education, lengthy-time period use of nonsteroidal anti-inflammatory pills).

Genetic reasons

Although maximum instances of AD are sporadic (i.e., now no longer inherited), familial varieties of AD do exist. Autosomal dominant AD, which debts for much less than 5% of instances, is sort of solely early onset AD; instances arise in at the least three people in 2 or greater generations, with 2 of the people being first-diploma spouse and children.

Familial clustering represents about 15–25% of past due-onset AD instances and most customarily entails past due-onset AD. In familial clustering, at the least 2 of the affected people are third-diploma spouse and children or closer.

Mutations within the following genes unequivocally reason early-onset autosomal dominant AD:

- The amyloid precursor protein (APP) gene on chromosome 21
- The presenilin-1 (PS1) gene on chromosome 14
- The presenilin-2 (PS2) gene on chromosome 1

All three of those genes cause a relative extra within the manufacturing of the stickier 42-amino acid shape of the Ab peptide over the much less sticky 40-amino-acid shape.

This beta-pleated peptide is postulated to have neurotoxic residences and to cause a cascade of events (as but incompletely understood) that consequences in neuronal loss of life, synapse loss, and the formation of NFTs and SPs, amongst different lesions. Nonetheless, the mutations which have been located to this point account for much less than 1/2 of of all instances of early-onset AD.

Other than the apolipoprotein E epsilon four (APOE E4) genotype, no polymorphisms in different genes were continually located to be related to past due-onset AD. However, genome-extensive affiliation research has diagnosed the subsequent extra susceptibility loci [40]:

- Clusterin (CLU) gene
- Phosphatidylinositol-binding clathrin meeting protein (PICALM) gene
- Complement receptor 1 (CR1) gene
- ATP-binding cassette sub-own circle of relatives A member 7 gene (ABCA7)
- Membrane-spanning gene cluster (MS4A6A/MS4A4E)
- Ephrin receptor A1 (EPHA1)
- CD33
- CD2AP

APP mutations

The remark that sufferers with Down syndrome (trisomy 21) increase cognitive deterioration and common pathological capabilities of AD with the aid of using center age brought about the invention of the APP gene on chromosome 21. Simultaneously, a locus segregating with a minority of early-onset familial AD kindred become mapped to this chromosome, within the identical place because the APP gene.

Subsequently, numerous missense mutations within the APP gene that ended in amino acid substitutions in APP had been diagnosed in those familial AD kindred. Such mutations seem to adjust the formerly defined proteolytic processing of APP, producing amyloidogenic varieties of Ab.

Skin fibroblasts from people wearing APP mutations produce extended Ab 42/43. Increased plasma awareness of Ab 42/43 is likewise visible in those sufferers, no matter age, sex, or medical popularity. Interestingly, a few sufferers with sporadic AD can also additionally showcase comparable elevations of plasma Ab 42/43.

PS1 and PS2 mutations

Approximately 50-70% of early-onset autosomal-dominant AD instances look like related to a locus (AD3) mapped with the aid of using genetic linkage to the lengthy arm of chromosome 14 (14q24.3). Numerous missense mutations were diagnosed on a robust candidate gene, referred to as PS1.

At the identical time, some other autosomal dominant locus answerable for early-onset AD become localized to chromosome 1. Two mutations had been diagnosed at the candidate gene, particular PS2. The physiological function of presenilins and the pathogenic results in their mutations aren't but nicely understood.

APOE

The gene encoding the cholesterol-wearing apolipoprotein E (APOE) on chromosome 19 has been connected to extended hazard for AD, basically past due-onset however additionally a few early-onset instances. The gene is inherited as an autosomal codominant trait with three alleles. The APOE E2 allele, the least widespread of the three not unusualplace APOE alleles, is related to the bottom hazard of growing AD, with a decrease charge of annual hippocampal atrophy and better cerebrospinal fluid Aβ and decrease phosphotau, suggesting much less AD pathology.

The E3 allele confers intermediate hazard of growing AD, with much less hazard than the E4 allele. The E3 allele, that is greater not unusualplace than the E2 allele, can also additionally guard tau from hyperphosphorylation, and the E2 allele's impact on tau phosphorylation is complex.

APOE E4 gene "dose" is correlated with extended hazard and in advance onset of AD. Individuals who're genetically predisposed to AD are suggested to intently manage their blood strain intently. Hypertension has been proven to have interaction with APOE E4 genotype to growth amyloid deposition in cognitively wholesome center-elderly and older adults; controlling high blood pressure can also additionally notably lower the hazard of growing amyloid deposits, even in people with genetic hazard.

Persons with 2 copies of the APOE E4 allele (four/four genotype) have a notably more hazard of growing AD than folks with different APOE subtypes. Mean age at onset is notably decrease within the presence of two APOE E4 copies. A collaborative observe has recommended that APOE E4 exerts its maximal impact earlier than the age of 70 years.

Many APOE E4 providers do now no longer increase AD, and plenty of sufferers with AD do now no longer have this allele. Therefore, the presence of an APOE E4 allele does now no longer stable the analysis of AD, however alternatively, the APOE E4 allele acts as a biologic hazard issue for the disorder, especially in the ones more youthful than 70 years.

According to at least one observe, publicity to particulate matter (PM) within the ambient air and its interactions with APOE alleles can also additionally make a contribution to the acceleration of mind growing old and the pathogenesis of AD. In addition to inspecting experimental mouse models, researchers analyzed facts on greater than three, six hundred US ladies among a long time of sixty-five and seventy-nine years from forty-eight states. None of the ladies had dementia while the observe started out. Data display that living in locations with first-rate PM exceeding EPA requirements extended the dangers for worldwide cognitive decline and all-reason dementia respectively with the aid of using 81 and 92%, with more potent destructive results in APOE ε4/four providers. These joint facts from human beings and mice offer the primary proof that neurodegenerative results of airborne PM can also additionally contain gene-surroundings interactions with APOE ε4.

Insulin resistance

A small observe with the aid of using Baker et al means that insulin resistance, as evidenced with the aid of using reduced cerebral glucose metabolic charge measured with the aid of using a particular form of positron emission tomography (PET) experiment, can be beneficial as an early marker of AD hazard, even earlier than the onset of MCI. The PET experiment discovered a qualitatively exclusive activation sample in sufferers with prediabetes or kind 2 diabetes mellitus all through a reminiscence encoding task, compared with wholesome those who had been now no longer insulin resistant.

Although the observe with the aid of using Baker et al had too few topics (n=23) for the consequences to attain statistical significance, an observe with the aid of using Schrijvers et al in a far large population (3,139 topics) located a comparable affiliation among insulin resistance and AD over three years, which then disappeared after that time. These researchers used an exclusive degree of insulin resistance, the homeostasis version assessment. Disturbances in insulin metabolism might not reason neurological adjustments however can also additionally have an effect on and boost up those adjustments, main to an in advance onset of AD.

Infection

A rising area of studies shows a huge affiliation among AD and persistent contamination with diverse species of spirochetes, together with the periodontal pathogen Treponemas and Borrelia burgdorferi, in addition to pathogens including herpes simplex virus kind 1. In vitro and animal research help the idea of contamination ensuing in persistent irritation and neuronal destruction. Ab has been proven to be an antimicrobial peptide, so its accumulation would possibly constitute a reaction to contamination.

Depression

Depression has been diagnosed as a hazard issue for AD and different dementias. Recent Framingham facts have helped bolster the epidemiological affiliation. The observe confirmed a 50% growth in AD and dementia in individuals who had been depressed at baseline. During a 17-12 months observe-up duration, a complete of 21.6% of members who had been depressed at baseline advanced dementia, compared with 16.6% of individuals who had been now no longer depressed.

In some other associated observe, recurrent despair become cited to be especially pernicious. One episode of despair conferred an 87–92% growth in dementia hazard, whilst having 2 or greater episodes almost doubled the hazard.

According to the consequences of a meta-evaluation of 23 population-primarily based totally, potential cohort research, past due-existence despair is related to an extended hazard for all-reason dementia, vascular dementia, and AD. The hazard for vascular dementia regarded to be notably better than the hazard for AD. The evaluation blanketed facts on sufferers 50 years and older who had been freed from dementia at baseline. The overall pattern blanketed within the pooled evaluation for all-reason dementia become 49,612 members, 5116 of whom had past due-existence despair.

Alternatively, a massive, longitudinal observe located that despair that begins offevolved early in existence will increase the hazard for AD. Researchers used facts from the Prospective Population Study of Women in Gothenburg Sweden, which started out in 1968. The observe pattern blanketed 800 ladies (imply age, forty-six years), born among 1914 and 1930, who had been observed up with in 1974, 1980, 1992, 2000, 2009, and 2012. Data display the ones ladies who skilled the onset of despair earlier than age two decades had been 3 instances much more likely to increase AD (adjusted HR, three.41; 95% CI, 1.78 - 6.54).

Head trauma

Moderate to intense head trauma has been documented as a hazard issue for the improvement of AD in addition to different varieties of dementia later in existence. Chen et al have proposed that annoying mind harm results in accumulation of amyloid precursor protein with its proteolytic enzymes at web sites of axonal harm, extended intracellular manufacturing of Ab, launch of Ab from injured axons into the extracellular space, and deposition of Ab into extracellular plaques.

An observe that observed over 7,000 US veterans of World War II confirmed that individuals who had sustained head accidents had two times the hazard of growing dementia later in existence, with veterans who suffered greater intense head trauma being at a good better hazard. The observe additionally located that the presence of the APOE gene and maintaining head trauma regarded to behave additively to growth the hazard of growing AD, even though there has been no direct correlation.

Epigenetics

Epigenetics is a extrade in gene expression that consequences from gene-surroundings interactions. This is mediated with the aid of using DNA methylation, RNA editing, and RNA interference without adjustments within the DNA sequence. Epigenetic factors in AD are recommended with the aid of using information that almost all of instances of AD are sporadic, arise in sufferers without a own circle of relatives records of the disorder, and feature onset past due in existence.

One environmental issue that has proven harm in laboratory animals regular with human AD is lead. Early publicity to steer in monkeys ended in plaque formation as they elderly. One component of early lead publicity seems to be extended oxidative strain in mind cells. Oxidative strain is the buildup of extra unfastened radicals that adjust methylation styles within the cells.

Early oxidative strain apart from lead has been postulated as one reason of sporadic AD. Brain cells in AD showcase overexpression and repression of AD genes, suggesting hypomethylation and hypermethylation, which can be related to oxidative strain.

Given that lead publicity to animals in childhood does now no longer produce manifestations till later in existence, persevered environmental strain can also additionally make a contribution to expression. Consequently, it's miles feasible that using antioxidant dietary supplements beginning in early life would possibly lower lengthy-time period oxidative strain and reduce the occurrence of AD. The paintings of Harman suggest that antioxidants can also additionally lower cellular harm and growing old with the aid of using reducing extra oxidative strain.

The handiest most important observe of 1 antioxidant, nutrition E, yielded disappointing consequences. However, the observe worried a totally confined time usage. At gift no different adjustments in environmental exposures were studied for prevention of AD, however this vicinity may be crucial in destiny lengthy-time period research.

Epidemiology

United States statistics

According to a 2017 record, AD influences a predicted 6.08 million human beings within the United States, and about 200,000 human beings more youthful than sixty-five years with AD represent the more youthful-onset US populace with AD. A large range of people have reduced cognitive feature (e.g., moderate cognitive impairment); this circumstance often evolves into complete-blown dementia, thereby growing the range of affected men and women. By the 12 months 2050, AD should have an effect on 13.8 million men and women within the United States.

Using information from Rochester, Minnesota, Genin et al calculated that on the age of eighty-five years, the lifetime hazard of AD without connection with APOE genotype became 11% in men and 14% in women; for APOE four/four companies, hazard ranged from 51% for men to 60% for women. For APOE three/four companies, hazard ranged from 23% for men to 30% for women. In French prevalence information, lifetime hazard for women at age eighty-five became 68% for APOE four/four companies and 35% for APOE three/four companies.

In the United States, AD is a main purpose of dying. While deaths from different foremost reasons were decreasing, deaths from of AD were growing. AD became the 6th main purpose of dying in 2017. Moreover, AD as an underlying purpose of dying is often underreported.

International statistics

Prevalence charges of AD just like the ones within the United States were suggested in industrialized nations. The incidence of dementia in men and women sixty-five years of age and older in North America is about 6-10%, with AD accounting for - thirds of those instances. If milder instances are included, the superiority charges double. Countries experiencing speedy will increase within the aged segments in their populace have charges drawing near the ones within the United States.

The World Health Organization's evaluation in 2000 at the Global Burden of Dementia, which became an integrative evaluation of forty-seven surveys throughout 17 countries, counseled that approximate charges for dementia from any purpose are beneath 1% in men and women elderly 60-sixty-nine years, growing to approximately 39% in men and women ninety-ninety-five years old. The incidence doubles with each five years of age inside that range, with few variations taking into consideration secular adjustments, age, gender, or location of living.

AD has end up almost two times as accepted as vascular dementia (VaD) in Korea, Japan, and China for the reason that early 1990s. American and European research always suggested AD to be extra accepted than VaD. The dementia incidence fee became located to be 11.2 in line with 1,000 amongst Chinese elderly 50 years and older at the islet of Kinmen. AD accounted for 64.6% and VaD for 29.3%. These effects, collectively with preceding research in Chinese populations, endorse that the charges of AD within the Chinese are low in comparison with the ones in whites.

In Nigeria, the superiority of dementia became located to be low. Indian research was contradictory, with each AD and VaD being extra accepted in extraordinary research.

Age distribution for Alzheimer sickness

The incidence of AD will increase with age. AD is maximum accepted in people older than 60 years. Some kinds of familial early-onset AD can seem as early because the 1/3 decade, however familial instances represent much less than 10% of AD typical.

More than ninety% of instances of AD are sporadic and arise in people older than 60 years. Of hobby, however, effects of a few research of nonagenarians and centenarians endorse that the hazard might also additionally lower in people older than ninety years. If so, age isn't always an unqualified hazard component for the sickness, however similarly look at of this be counted is needed.

Savva et al located that within the aged populace, the affiliation among dementia and the pathological functions of AD (e.g., neuritic plaques, diffuse plaques, tangles) is more potent in men and women seventy-five years of age than in men and women ninety-five years of age. These effects had been finished through assessing 456 brains donated to the populace-primarily based totally Medical Research Council Cognitive Function and Ageing Study from men and women sixty-nine-103 years of age at dying.

Studies have validated that the connection among cerebral atrophy and dementia persist into the oldest a long time however that the electricity of affiliation among pathological functions of AD and medical dementia diminishes. It is essential to take age into consideration whilst assessing the probably impact of interventions towards dementia.

Sexual variations in prevalence

Some research has suggested a better hazard of AD in girls than in guys; different research, however, together with the Aging, Demographics, and Memory Study, located no distinction in hazard among guys and girls. Almost thirds of Americans with AD are girls. Among AD sufferers typical, any sexual disparity might also additionally virtually replicate girls' better existence expectancy. Among folks that are heterozygous for the APOE E4 allele, however, Payami et al located a twofold multiplied hazard in girls.

Race-associated variations in prevalence

AD and different dementias are extra not unusualplace in African Americans than in whites. According to the Alzheimer's Association, within the populace elderly seventy one years and older, African Americans are nearly two times as probably to have AD and different dementias as whites (21.3% of African Americans vs 11.2% of whites). The range of Hispanic sufferers studied on this age institution became too small to decide the superiority of dementia on this populace.

Based on information for Medicare beneficiaries age sixty five and older, 6.9% of whites, 9.4% of African Americans, and 11.5% of Hispanics have AD or different dementias, and the superiority of AD and different dementias is better in older age groups.

In a look at of 1255 human beings, together with each African American (N=173) and Caucasian participants, researchers located that cerebrospinal fluid from African Americans tended to include decrease degrees of mind protein tau, a biomarker related to AD. However, this did now no longer appear to defend them from the sickness; they had been simply as probably as Caucasians to be cognitively impaired on this look at. These effects endorse that evaluation of biomarkers for AD ought to be adjusted for race.

Prognosis

AD is to start with related to reminiscence impairment that step by step worsens. Over time, sufferers with AD also can show anxiety, despair, insomnia, agitation, and paranoia. As their sickness progresses, sufferers with AD come to require help with simple sports of each day living, together with dressing, bathing, and toileting. Eventually, problems with strolling and swallowing might also additionally expand. Feeding can be viable simplest through gastrointestinal tube, and problem swallowing might also additionally cause aspiration pneumonia.

The time from prognosis to dying varies from as low as three years to so long as 10 or extra years. Patients with early-onset AD have a tendency to have an extra competitive, speedy path than people with past due-onset AD. The number one purpose of dying is intercurrent infection, including pneumonia.

Patient Education

When counseling sufferers following a prognosis of AD, it's miles vital to contain the affected person's own circle of relatives and others who will play a assisting position within the discussion. It is essential to emphasize that now no longer simplest the affected person however additionally folks that help the sufferers will probably revel in reactions of unhappiness and anger and that those are regular reactions to this type of prognosis.

As the affected person's signs end up extra reported, a talk should be opened concerning the affected person's needs for care whilst she or he is now no longer capable of make the essential choices. Durable energy of legal professional ought to be discussed, with specific interest to who will make selections for each clinical and economic problems. Medical boost directives ought to be taken into consideration whilst the affected person continues to be capin a position to take part within the decision-making process.

Throughout the path of the sickness, own circle of relative's contributors ought to be cautious to choose certified and sincere people to be concerned within the daily control of the affected person. Caregivers want to stability interest to the affected person's bodily desires with keeping admire for the affected person as a able grownup, to the volume allowed through the development of the sickness. Any suspicions of elder abuse ought to be right now addressed.

Above all, counseling of AD sufferers and households ought to emphasize that sufferers ought to preserve to have interaction in sports that they experience doing. Maintaining a top-quality great of existence is key.

The following assets can be useful to percentage with sufferers and their households:

- MedlinePlus -Alzheimer's Disease
- The National Institute on Aging -General Information on Alzheimer's Disease
- Caring for Someone with Alzheimer's (video collection)
- The National Alzheimer's Association

Alzheimer Disease Clinical Presentation

History

Patients with Alzheimer sickness (AD) maximum normally gift with insidiously innovative reminiscence loss, to which different spheres of cognition are impaired over numerous years. This loss can be related to slowly innovative behavioral adjustments. After reminiscence loss happens, sufferers may additionally revel in language issues (e.g., anomic aphasia or anomia) and impairment of their visuospatial competencies and govt functions.

Patients with moderate AD generally have relatively much less apparent govt, language, and/or visuospatial disorder. In strange displays, disorder in cognitive domain names aside from reminiscence can be maximum apparent. In later tiers, many sufferers expand extrapyramidal disorder together with akathisia, parkinsonism, dystonia, bradykinesia, tremor, and tardive dyskinesia.

Substantially much less not unusualplace, however biopsy or post-mortem-proven, displays consist of proper parietal lobe syndrome, innovative aphasia, spastic paraparesis, and impaired visuospatial competencies, that is subsumed beneath the visible version of AD.

It is essential to attain an entire record now no longer simplest from the affected person however additionally from a person who is aware of the affected person properly. In addition, an own circle of relatives records of AD or different kinds of dementia ought to be noted.

Here are a few key factors to maintain in thoughts whilst taking records of an affected person with suspected AD:

- Many sufferers with AD lack perception into impairments and can even deny deficits.
- Early within the path of AD, sufferers might also additionally have preserved perception into the path in their sickness with preserved social and occupational functioning.

- It is essential to represent the onset and early signs to distinguish different pathologies which might be extra abrupt, including vascular dementia.
- Obtaining a great evaluation of the affected person's purposeful skills frequently is aided through an informed informant.

One might also additionally divide purposeful skills into simple and instrumental sports of each day living (ADLs). Basic ADLs (BADLs) consist of sports for self-mantainence including grooming, while instrumental ADLs (IADLs) are extra complicated obligations including paying bills.

Physical Examination

At the time of preliminary prognosis, an entire bodily exam, together with an in depth neurologic exam and an intellectual popularity exam, ought to be executed to assess sickness level and rule out comorbid situations. Initial intellectual popularity trying out ought to consist of assessment of the subsequent:

- Attention and concentration
- Recent and far off reminiscence
- Language
- Praxis (ie, capacity to carry out professional motor obligations without nonverbal prompting)
- Executive feature
- Visuospatial feature

Cognitive functions of early AD consist of reminiscence loss, moderate anomic aphasia, and visuospatial disorder. At all next observe-up visits, a complete intellectual popularity exam ought to be executed to assess sickness development and become aware of the improvement of any new neuropsychiatric signs.

Brief standardized examinations, including the Mini-Mental Status Examination (MMSE), are much less touchy and precise than longer batteries which might be mainly tailor-made to person sufferers. Other examples consist of the Montreal Cognitive Assessment (MoCA) and the Saint Louis University Mental Status (SLUMS) exam. Nonetheless, screening assessments have a position, especially as a baseline. For extra data, see the Medscape Reference article Screening for Cognitive Impairment.

An entire neurologic exam is executed to search for symptoms and symptoms of different illnesses that might purpose dementia, including Parkinson sickness or more than one strokes. In sufferers with AD, the neurologic examination is typically regular however might also additionally monitor minor abnormalities including hyposmia or anosmia.

Stages of Alzheimer Disease

AD may be categorized into the subsequent tiers:

- Preclinical
- Mild
- Moderate

- Severe

Preclinical Alzheimer sickness

The pathologic adjustments related to AD start within the entorhinal cortex, that is close to the hippocampus and without delay linked to it. AD then proceeds to the hippocampus, that is the shape this is vital to the formation of quick-time period and lengthy-time period memories. Affected areas start to atrophy. These mind adjustments arise a long time earlier than any symptoms and symptoms or signs seem.

Memory loss, the primary seen sign, is the principle characteristic of amnestic moderate cognitive impairment (MCI). Many scientists suppose MCI is frequently a preliminary, transitional medical segment among regular mind growing older and AD. For extra data, see the Medscape Reference article Mild Cognitive Impairment.

An affected person with preclinical AD might also additionally seem absolutely regular on bodily exam and intellectual popularity trying out. At this level, there's generally no alteration in judgment or the capacity to carry out sports of each day living.

Mild Alzheimer sickness

As AD starts offevolved to have an effect on the cerebral cortex, reminiscence loss maintains and impairment of different cognitive skills emerges. This level is called moderate AD. The medical prognosis of AD is generally made at some point of this level. Signs of moderate AD can consist of the subsequent:

- Memory loss
- Confusion approximately the region of acquainted locations (getting misplaced starts offevolved to arise)
- Taking longer to perform regular each day obligations
- Trouble dealing with cash and paying bills
- Compromised judgment frequently main to horrific selections
- Loss of spontaneity and feel of initiative

- Mood and character adjustments; multiplied anxiety

The developing range of plaques and tangles first harm regions of the mind that manage reminiscence, language, and reasoning (see the photos below). Later within the sickness, bodily skills decline. This ends in a state of affairs in moderate AD wherein someone appears to be wholesome however is genuinely having increasingly more problem making feel of the arena round him or her. The recognition that something is inaccurate frequently comes steadily due to the fact the early symptoms and symptoms may be pressured with adjustments that could show up generally with growing older.

Acknowledging those symptoms and symptoms of AD and figuring out to are looking for diagnostic trying out may be a hurdle for sufferers and their households to cross. In many instances, the own circle of relatives has a extra tough time dealing with the prognosis than the affected person does, in all likelihood due to apathy from the AD. Following the preliminary prognosis, sufferers ought to be cautiously monitored for depressed temper. Although it's miles not unusualplace for sufferers with early AD to be depressed approximately the prognosis, they hardly ever end up suicidal.

Moderate Alzheimer sickness

By the time AD reaches the slight level, harm has unfolded similarly to the regions of the cerebral cortex that manage language, reasoning, sensory processing, and aware thought. Affected areas preserve to atrophy, and symptoms and symptoms and signs of the sickness end up extra reported and tremendous. Behavior issues, including wandering and agitation, can arise. More in depth supervision and care end up essential, and this may be tough for lots spouses and households.

The signs of this level can consist of the subsequent:

- Increasing reminiscence loss and confusion
- Shortened interest span
- Problems spotting pals and own circle of relative's contributors

- Difficulty with language; issues with reading, writing, operating with numbers
- Difficulty organizing mind and wondering logically
- Inability to study new matters or to deal with new or surprising situations
- Restlessness, agitation, anxiety, tearfulness, wandering, particularly within the past due afternoon or at night
- Repetitive statements or motion; occasional muscle twitches
- Hallucinations, delusions, suspiciousness or paranoia, irritability
- Loss of impulse manage (proven via conduct including undressing at irrelevant instances or locations or vulgar language)
- Perceptual-motor issues (including problem getting out of a chair or putting the table)

Behavior is the end result of complicated mind approaches, all of which take location in a fragment of a 2d within the wholesome mind. In AD, lots of those approaches are disturbed, and that is the premise for lots distressing or irrelevant behaviors. For example, sufferers might also additionally angrily refuse to take a tub or dress due to the fact they do now no longer apprehend what the caregiver has requested them to do. If they do apprehend, they'll now no longer keep in mind a way to do what became requested.

This anger is a masks for underlying confusion and anxiety. Consequently, the hazard for violent and homicidal conduct is maximum at this level of sickness development. Patients ought to be cautiously monitored for any conduct which could compromise the protection of these round them.

For someone who can't keep in mind the beyond or assume the destiny, the arena round them may be peculiar and frightening. Staying near a relied on and acquainted caregiver can be the simplest aspect that makes feel and gives security. A man or woman with AD might also additionally continuously observe his or her caregiver and be troubled whilst the man or woman is out of sight.

Judgment and impulse manage preserve to say no at this level. For example, commencing garments might also additionally appear affordable to someone with AD who feels warm and does now no longer apprehend or keep in mind that undressing in public isn't always acceptable.

Severe Alzheimer sickness

In the closing level, intense AD, plaques and tangles are tremendous at some stage in the mind, and regions of the mind have atrophied similarly. Patients can't apprehend own circle of relatives and cherished ones or talk in any way. They are absolutely depending on others for care. All feel of self appears to vanish.

Other signs can consist of the subsequent:

- Weight loss
- Seizures, pores and skin infections, problem swallowing
- Groaning, moaning, or grunting
- Increased sleeping

- Lack of bladder and bowel manage

In cease-level AD, sufferers can be in mattress a lot or all the time. Death is frequently the end result of different ailments, often aspiration pneumonia.

Dementia in Motor Neuron Disease

Overview

Patients with motor neuron sickness (MND) are typically freed from cognitive impairment, however proof is developing to help an affiliation among MND and frontal lobe or frontotemporal dementia (FTD).

MND, because the call shows, is a natural motor disease with none full-size proof of sensory signs, extraocular motion disturbances, bladder and bowel disorder, or cognitive impairment. Cognitive impairment in amyotrophic lateral sclerosis (ALS) is correlated with pathologic and radiographic adjustments within the cerebral cortex past the motor areas. Evidence of impairment can clinically be visible in nearly 1/2 of sufferers via direct neuropsychological trying out, however frank FTD happens in a constrained percent of sufferers.

Some recommend that frontotemporal lobe dementia with motor neuron sickness (FTD/MND) is nosologically awesome; others endorse that it's miles a part of a spectrum of illnesses encompassing conventional MND at one cease and FTD at the opposite.

The discovery of pathologic transactive reaction deoxyribonucleic acid (DNA) binding protein forty-three (TDP-forty-three) in ALS and FTD with ubiquitinated inclusions confirms that those are intently associated situations belonging to a brand new biochemical elegance of neurodegenerative illnesses, the TDP-forty three proteinopathies.

Complications

Complications in FTD/MND can consist of the subsequent:

- Progressive bulbar palsy effects in dysphagia, the hazard of aspiration pneumonia, and mutism
- Muscular losing and weak spot might also additionally arise
- Parkinsonism might also additionally expand in a few sufferers
- Dyspnea and hypoxic encephalopathy can be associated positionally and may intervene with reclining for sleep

Prognosis

Progressive dementia with signs of govt disorder, character extrade, and motor weak spot ends in intense morbidity. Death generally happens inside three years of onset from inanition, pulmonary failure, and aspiration.

Patients with FTD/MND typically observe an extra speedy path than do sufferers with both FTD or MND by myself. They are much more likely to have a bulbar shape of MND, which might also additionally assist to give an explanation for its extra competitive path.

Treatment considerations

Treatment techniques for FTD might also additionally follow to FTD/MND, however this isn't always recognized for certain. Current remedies specifically are supportive and directed towards the functions of MND.

Evaluate and deal with sialorrhea, impaired breathing, swallowing, and mobility. There isn't any surgical remedy for FTD/MND, however recollect gastrostomy tube feeding for sufferers with intense bulbar signs, intense dysphagia, and comparatively moderate dementia and limb weak spot. Prior to gastrostomy, automatically gentle diets may be tried. [#TreatmentDiet]

Consider neuroprotective agents (e.g., riluzole, gabapentin) or dietary supplements (e.g., creatine) to hold muscle bulk, however be aware that their efficacy in FTD/MND is even extra unsure than its miles in MND.

Depending at the affected person's career and stage of cognitive and neurologic disorder, clinical go away of absence or early retirement can be advisable.

Patient training

For affected person training data, see the Brain and Nervous System Center, in addition to Dementia Overview, Dementia Medication Overview, and Dementia in Amyotrophic Lateral Sclerosis (Lou Gehrig's Disease).

Etiology

Worldwide, frontotemporal lobe dementia with motor neuron sickness (FTD/MND) is a sporadic circumstance with an unknown etiology. It is characterized through pyramidal mobileular loss within the frontal and temporal lobes and degeneration of motor neurons within the hypoglossal nucleus and spinal motor neurons. Pyramidal neurons withinthe premotor cortex generally are preserved.

Takeda et al have proven that ALS pathology initiated through cytoplasmic inclusions and neuronal loss in layer II-III of the transentorhinal cortex (TEC)–molecular dentate gyrus (DG) projection and subiculum is precise to ALS. This isn't like the neurofibrillary tangles of Alzheimer sickness, dominant in layer II-III of the entorhinal cortex. This might also additionally offer a foundation for medical characterization of reminiscence deficits of ALS, which can be awesome from the ones of Alzheimer sickness.

TDP-forty-three has been recognized because the foremost pathologic protein in sporadic ALS and has additionally been located within the maximum not unusualplace pathologic subtype of FTD (i.e., frontotemporal lobar degeneration with ubiquitinated inclusions). Data now endorse that delocalization, accumulation, and ubiquitination of TDP-forty three within the cytoplasm of motor neurons are early dysfunctions within the cascade of the occasions main to motor neuron degeneration in ALS.

Signs and signs replicate frontal and temporal lobe disorder with decrease motor neuron–kind weak spot, muscle atrophy, and fasciculations.

Genetics

A minority of sufferers have a own circle of relatives records of FTD/MND, however this overlap syndrome can be associated with different neurodegenerative overlap syndromes that consist of variable levels of dementia, MND, and parkinsonism.

The maximum not unusualplace mutation, accounting for 10% of all Western hemisphere ALS, is a hexanucleotide repeat enlargement in C9orf72. This and numerous different genes implicate altered RNA processing and protein-degradation pathways withinside the middle of ALS pathogenesis. The nomenclature MSP1, MSP2, and MSP3 can be used for VCP-, HNRNPA2B1-, and HNRNPA1-related sickness, respectively. Potential relevance has been proven concerning the pathobiology of extra not unusualplace MNDs including ALS, imparting a further hyperlink among ALS and FTD.

Two of the genes inflicting FTD by myself (CHMP2B and GRN) are related to a broken autophagy/lysosomal pathway. However, the 1/3 FTD gene (MAPT) maps to an extraordinary pathway, which possibly isn't always surprising, seeing that it's miles related to an extraordinary (now no longer p62-associated) mind pathology. Wang et al currently located courting among sporadic kinds of Alzheimer-kind dementia and ALS this is connected to I2(PP2A) and the ability of I2(PP2A)-primarily based totally therapeutics for those illnesses.

Ubiquilin-2 mouse fashions offer treasured equipment for figuring out the mechanisms underlying ALS-FTD pathogenesis and for investigating healing techniques to terminate sickness.

C9orf72 repeat enlargement has been recognized as an essential genetic hazard component for each motor neuron sickness and frontotemporal dementia.

This has helped to verify that the sickness bureaucracy a part of a spectrum of primary neurodegenerative approaches.

Overall, the modern-day kingdom of information factors to not unusualplace mechanisms chargeable for susceptibilities precise to neuronal classes.

Epidemiology

Occurrence within the United States

Frontal lobe dementia is the second one or 1/3 maximum not unusualplace kind of degenerative dementia in post-mortem collection. The particular frequency with which frontotemporal lobe dementia with motor neuron sickness (FTD/MND) happens in post-mortem or populace research is unknown (however low).

International occurrence

In a Scandinavian post-mortem collection, dementia became suggested in 2-6% of sufferers with MND. The relative frequency of FTD/MND in all sufferers with dementia seems comparable within the United States and Japan. Certain populations (e.g., Chamorro Indians of Guam, indigenous citizens of the Kii Peninsula) have a disproportionately better prevalence and incidence of overlap degenerative syndromes (MND, dementia, parkinsonism).

Race-, sex-, and age-associated demographics

FTD/MND has been defined in sufferers of Asian, European, and African descent. No information is to be had approximately prevalence and incidence amongst racial groups.

Men look like affected barely extra often than girls, however this distinction might not be full-size. The suggest age of onset in sporadic instances varies amongst collection however typical is 55-sixty-five years. Familial instances have a tendency to be more youthful.

Patient History

Frontotemporal lobe dementia with motor neuron sickness (FTD/MND) generally gives as a extrade in character with deterioration in social conduct. Initial behavioral adjustments range however consist of abulia, apathy, and decreased spontaneity and/or initiation. Some sufferers end up strikingly disinhibited, overactive, and admittedly irrelevant, with emotional lability. With sickness development, however, even the ones sufferers manifesting disinhibition and restlessness end up more and more apathetic.

Stereotypic conduct and repetitive rituals of hoarding, dressing, wandering, and toileting may be found. In addition, sufferers might also additionally overeat, show off hyperoral tendencies, and expand meals fads (even though that is extra exceptional). Some sufferers might also additionally maintain meals of their mouth for extended durations without swallowing.

Dynamic, spontaneous speech output step by step declines, ensuing in anarthria and mutism. A subset of sufferers gives with hastily innovative aphasia. Despite development to anarthria, post-mortem research display that anarthria can arise within the absence of full-size involvement of the hypoglossal nucleus. Although there's full-size reminiscence impairment, this isn't always as distinguishing because the frontal lobe or language functions.

Posterior cortical functions (e.g., visuospatial competencies) are preserved and/or spared till the preterminal tiers.

The medical sample displays the topographic sample of atrophy, frequently seen radiographically, with asymmetrical frontotemporal atrophy. If asymmetrically worse within the left (language-dominant) hemisphere, aphasia is a possible and distinguished medical characteristic.

Throughout the path of the sickness, symptoms and symptoms and signs of MND additionally development. Cognitive adjustments frequently precede symptoms and symptoms of MND. Limb weak spot and dysphagia in the end up disabling, even though a few sufferers have a on the whole bulbar sample of weak spot with relative sparing of limb electricity.

Consensus medical standards detailing middle and supportive functions for FTD syndromes were published.

Physical Examination

Patients with frontotemporal lobe dementia with motor neuron sickness (FTD/MND) generally carry out poorly on checks of frontal lobe feature (i.e., Wisconsin card sorting, photo sequencing, verbal fluency checks). Memory is impaired, however much less always within the moderate tiers.

Clinical symptoms and symptoms of MND generally observe or accompany dementia onset. MND symptoms and symptoms consist of bulbar weak spot with dysarthria and dysphagia, limb weak spot, muscle losing and fasciculations, and, of finest concern, dyspnea.

Akinesia and pressure are unusual on this disease however extra not unusualplace in sufferers with an extended c programming language among onset of dementia and neurologic symptoms and symptoms (extra than 24mo in a Japanese collection). This might also additionally replicate, in part, the variable involvement of the substantia nigra and different pigmented brainstem nuclei which might be found in kind of 50% of sufferers at post-mortem. This, in turn, might also additionally range among populations (extra not unusualplace in Chamorro Indians).

Moon et al have proven that sluggish vertical saccades are not unusualplace in FTD/MND. This might also additionally require extra research within the destiny to verify the involvement of the burst neurons within the dorsal midbrain in sufferers with FTD/MND.

Diagnostic Considerations

Conditions to recollect within the differential prognosis of frontotemporal lobe dementia with motor neuron sickness (FTD/MND) consist of the subsequent:

- Alzheimer sickness
- ALS
- Dementia with Lewy bodies
- Frontal and temporal lobe dementia
- Frontal lobe syndromes
- Pick sickness
- Vascular dementia
- Dementia in Parkinson sickness
- Creutzfeldt-Jakob sickness

Imaging Studies

Computed tomography (CT) scanning in sufferers with frontotemporal lobe dementia with motor neuron sickness (FTD/MND) might also additionally display moderate, generalized cerebral atrophy or asymmetrical frontotemporal atrophy.

Because it gives more decision than CT scanning does, magnetic resonance imaging (MRI) might also additionally monitor selective frontal and anterior temporal atrophy that can't be favored on CT scanning.

Single-photon emission CT (SPECT) scanning frequently demonstrates decreased blood go with the drift in an asymmetrical, frontotemporal sample.

In a current look at, it's been proven that lack of grey be counted extent in motor and extramotor areas of simplest ALS sufferers with FTD and now no longer of

ALS sufferers without FTD shows awesome websites of important pathology. This may additionally offer a few thoughts approximately sickness onset. Brain volumetric measures supplemented through histopathological correlations and different neuroimaging techniques, including diffusion tensor imaging, might also additionally offer perception into ALS pathophysiology.

A look at suggested that glucose hypometabolism on positron emission tomography (PET) scans in sufferers with dementia related to MND affected simplest the frontal lobes, sparing the temporal lobes. This contrasted with frontotemporal dementia, wherein glucose hypometabolism is visible within the frontal lobes and temporal lobes. In Alzheimer sickness, PET scans might also additionally monitor glucose hypometabolism within the parietal and temporal areas bilaterally.

Boyajian et al endorsed magnetoencephalography (MEG) as an effective new device for studying the contribution of cortical disorder to motor disability, which could represent the sickness process.

Histologic Findings

Early within the sickness, frontotemporal lobe dementia with motor neuron sickness (FTD/MND) preferentially influences frontal and temporal lobes, the hypoglossal nucleus, and the spinal motor neurons. The later and terminal tiers monitor histologic proof of tremendous cortical involvement. In the frontal and temporal lobes, microscopic adjustments consist of lack of pyramidal cells, spongiform neuropil extrade, and astrocytic gliosis.

Ubiquitinated, tau-poor inclusions are gift within side the frontal cortex and the dentate gyrus of the hippocampus. Pick cells (inflated neurons) and Pick bodies (ubiquitin and tau-high-quality intracellular inclusions) are absent. Betz cells within the precentral gyrus generally are affected.

In about 50% of sufferers, neuronal loss and pigmentary incontinence within the substantia nigra and different pigmented brainstem neurons arise, even in sufferers without clinically overt parkinsonism. There may be marked hypoglossal and spinal motor neuron degeneration (even though this isn't always vital for sufferers to development to an anarthric kingdom) and ubiquitinated tau-poor inclusions within the spinal neurons.

Additional Studies

The following research also are used within the assessment of sufferers with frontotemporal lobe dementia with motor neuron sickness (FTD/MND):

- Typical blood research
- Thyroid feature checks
- Vitamin B-12 and folate degrees

Venereal Disease Research Laboratory test

The electroencephalogram can continue to be regular even within the later tiers of dementia, however frequently, moderate dysrhythmic slowing happens this is every so often asymmetrical.

Electromyography might also additionally reveal tremendous denervation in limb muscles. Early within the sickness, particularly in sufferers with a predominantly bulbar onset, findings might not satisfy the Lambert or El Escorial standards for motor neuron sickness.

Pharmacologic Considerations

No precise remedy is to be had for frontotemporal lobe dementia with motor neuron sickness (FTD/MND). Treatments for MND, including riluzole, do now no longer seem to have an effect on the path of the dementia-inducing infection. Riluzole is presently the simplest certified medicine for MND. Available information from healing trials in MND do now no longer display useful cognitive effects, even though there aren't any precise contraindications on this context.

Gabapentin has been studied in trials as a sickness-enhancing agent in sufferers with MND however does now no longer reveal precise cognitive-improving properties.

Acetylcholinesterase inhibitors (e.g., donepezil, rivastigmine) are used to accurate the cholinergic impact related to Alzheimer sickness. Although now no longer studied mainly in FTD, anecdotal reviews endorse they'll growth irritability in sufferers with FTD.

Patients with FTD who've profound presynaptic serotonergic deficits and behavioral disturbances might also additionally reply to selective serotonin reuptake inhibitors.

Optimal symptomatic dopaminergic remedy ought to be supplied to sufferers with overlap syndromes with idiopathic Parkinson sickness and MND. On the opposite hand, selective dopamine blockers, including olanzapine, can be beneficial in agitated sufferers;

reveal for unfavorable effects, including extrapyramidal syndromes.

Depression

Practice Essentials

Major depressive disease has full-size ability morbidity and mortality, contributing to suicide, prevalence and unfavorable results of clinical infection, disruption in interpersonal relationships, substance abuse, and misplaced paintings time. According to the CDC, in 2019, 2.8% of adults skilled intense signs of despair, 4.2% skilled slight signs, and 11.5% skilled moderate signs within the beyond 2 weeks. The percent of adults who skilled any signs of despair became maximum amongst the ones elderly 18–29 years (21.0%), accompanied through the ones elderly 45–64 years (18.4%) and sixty-five and older (18.4%), and lastly, through the ones elderly 30–44 years (16.8%). Women had been much more likely than guys to revel in moderate, slight, or intense signs of despair. With suitable remedy, 70–80% of people with foremost depressive disease can reap a full-size discount in signs.

Signs and signs

Most sufferers with foremost depressive disease gift with a regular appearance. In sufferers with extra intense signs, a decline in grooming and hygiene can be found, in addition to a extrade in weight. Patients may additionally display the subsequent:

Psychomotor retardation

Flattening or lack of reactivity within the affected persons have an effect on (i.e., emotional expression)

Psychomotor agitation or restlessness

Major depressive disease

Among the standards for a primary depressive disease, at the least five of the subsequent signs should were gift at some point of the identical 2-week period (and at the least 1 of the signs should be dwindled hobby/pride or depressed temper):

- **Depressed temper:** For kids and youth, this may additionally be an irritable temper
- Diminished hobby or lack of pride in nearly all sports (anhedonia)
- Significant weight extrade or urge for food disturbance: For kids, this may be failure to reap anticipated weight gain
- Sleep disturbance (insomnia or hypersomnia)
- Psychomotor agitation or retardation
- Fatigue or lack of energy
- Feelings of worthlessness
- Diminished capacity to suppose or concentrate; indecisiveness
- Recurrent mind of dying, recurrent suicidal ideation without a particular plan, or a suicide strive or precise plan for committing suicide

Diagnosis

Screening gadgets

Self-record screening gadgets for despair consist of the subsequent:

- **Patient Health Questionnaire-9 (PHQ-9):** A 9-object despair scale; every object is scored from 0-three, imparting a 0-27 severity rating.
- **Beck Depression Inventory (BDI) or the Beck Depression Inventory-II (BDI-II):** 21-query symptom-score scales imparting a 0-63 severity rating.
- **BDI for number one care:** A 7-query scale tailored from the BDI.
- **Zung Self-Rating Depression Scale:** A 20-object survey.

- **Center for Epidemiologic Studies-Depression Scale (CES-D):** A 20-object tool that lets in sufferers to assess their feelings, conduct, and outlook from the preceding week.

In assessment to the above self-record scales, the Hamilton Depression Rating Scale (HDRS) is executed through an educated expert, now no longer the affected person. The HDRS has 17 or 21 items, scored from 0-2 or 0-four; a complete rating of 0-7 is taken into consideration regular, whilst ratings of 20 or better suggest reasonably intense despair.

The Geriatric Depression Scale (GDS), even though evolved for older adults, has additionally been proven in more youthful adults. The GDS incorporates 30 items; a quick-shape GDS has 15 items.

Laboratory research

No diagnostic laboratory checks are to be had to diagnose foremost depressive disease, however targeted laboratory research can be beneficial to exclude ability clinical ailments which could gift as foremost depressive disease.

Management

In all affected person populations, the aggregate of medicine and psychotherapy typically gives the fastest and maximum sustained reaction.

Pharmacotherapy

Drugs used for remedy of despair consist of the subsequent:

- Selective serotonin reuptake inhibitors (SSRIs)
- Serotonin/norepinephrine reuptake inhibitors (SNRIs)
- Atypical antidepressants
- Tricyclic antidepressants (TCAs)
- Monoamine oxidase inhibitors (MAOIs)
- N-Methyl-D-aspartate (NMDA) receptor antagonists
- St. John's wort (Hypericum perforatum)

Psychotherapy

There are some of proof-primarily based totally psychotherapeutic remedies for adults with foremost depressive disease. The following were deemed to have robust studies help through Division 12 of the American Psychological Association:

- Behavior Therapy/Behavioral Activation
- Cognitive Therapy

- Cognitive Behavioral Analysis System of Psychotherapy
- Interpersonal psychotherapy (IPT)
- Problem-fixing remedy (PST)

Self-Management/Self-Control Therapy

Evidence-primarily based totally psychotherapeutic remedies for kids and youth with foremost depressive disease consist of the subsequent:

- Interpersonal psychotherapy (IPT)
- Cognitive-behavioral remedy (CBT)
- Behavior remedy (BT)

Many of those remedies comprise a parent/own circle of relatives thing whilst operating with kids or youth.

In moderate instances, psychosocial interventions are frequently endorsed as first-line remedies. The American Psychiatric Association (APA) tenet helps this method however notes that combining psychotherapy with antidepressant medicine can be extra suitable for sufferers with slight to intense foremost depressive disease.

Electroconvulsive remedy

Electroconvulsive remedy (ECT) is a noticeably powerful remedy for despair. The indicators for ECT consist of the subsequent:

- Need for a speedy antidepressant reaction
- Failure of drug therapies
- History of top reaction to ECT
- Patient preference
- High hazard of suicide
- High hazard of clinical morbidity and mortality

Stimulation techniques

Transcranial magnetic stimulation (TMS) is accepted through the FDA for remedy-resistant foremost despair.

Vagus nerve stimulation (VNS) has been accepted through the FDA to be used in grownup sufferers who've didn't reply to at the least four good enough medicine and/or ECT remedy regimens. The stimulation tool calls for surgical implantation.

Background

As many as thirds of human beings with despair do now no longer understand that they have got a treatable infection and consequently do now no longer are looking for expert assist. In addition, chronic lack of information and misperceptions of the sickness through the public, together with many fitness providers, as a private weak spot or failing that may be willed or wanted away ends in painful stigmatization and avoidance of the prognosis through lots of the ones affected.

In the number one care putting, wherein lots of those sufferers first are looking for remedy, the providing proceedings frequently may be somatic, including fatigue, headache, stomach distress, or sleep issues.

The American Psychiatric Association's Diagnostic Statistical Manual of Mental Disorders, Fifth Edition, Text Revision (DSM-five-TR) classifies the depressive issues as disruptive temper dysregulation disease, foremost depressive disease (together with foremost depressive episode), chronic depressive disease (dysthymia), premenstrual dysphoric disease, and depressive disease because of some other clinical circumstance. In addition, depressive issues can be similarly labeled through specifiers that consist of peripartum onset, seasonal sample, melancholic functions, temper-congruent or temper-incongruent psychotic functions, traumatic distress, and catatonia. The not unsualplace characteristic of the depressive issues is the presence of sad, empty, or irritable temper, observed through somatic and cognitive adjustments that substantially have an effect on the person's capability to feature. What differs amongst them are problems of duration, timing, or presumed etiology.

The differential prognosis for despair consists of different psychiatric issues, CNS illnesses, endocrine issues, drug-associated situations, infectious and inflammatory illnesses, and sleep-associated issues.

Depression screening checks may be used to display for despair and bipolar disease. The maximum extensively used is the Patient Health Questionnaire-9 (PHQ-9). It is essential to apprehend that the effects acquired from using any despair score scales are imperfect in any populace, particularly the geriatric populace.

Many powerful remedies are to be had for foremost depressive disease, together with psychotherapy (e.g., cognitive-behavioral remedy, interpersonal psychotherapy, conduct remedy), used both by myself or in aggregate with medicine. However, the mixed method gives a few sufferers with the fastest and maximum sustained reaction. Uncomplicated despair that isn't always intense normally responds similarly properly to psychotherapy or an antidepressant.

There is proof to help using all antidepressants accepted through the FDA to be used in foremost despair, even though predicting what a person affected person's reaction to a selected agent might be is tough. Assuming adherence to the remedy routine and absence of drug or sickness-kingdom interactions, remedy for 2–12 weeks at a healing-dose stage is generally had to reap a medical reaction. The desire of medicine ought to be guided through predicted protection and tolerability, doctor familiarity, and private and own circle of relatives records of preceding remedies.

Pathophysiology

The underlying pathophysiology of foremost depressive disease has now no longer been truly defined. Current proof factors to a complicated interplay among neurotransmitter availability and receptor law and sensitivity underlying the affective signs.

Clinical and preclinical trials endorse a disturbance in primary apprehensive device serotonin (five-HT) hobby as an essential component. Other neurotransmitters implicated consist of norepinephrine (NE), dopamine (DA), glutamate, and mind-derived neurotrophic component (BDNF). However, pills that produce simplest an acute upward thrust in neurotransmitter availability, including cocaine or amphetamines, do now no longer have the efficacy over the years that antidepressants do.

The position of CNS five-HT hobby within the pathophysiology of foremost depressive disease is recommended through the healing efficacy of selective serotonin reuptake inhibitors (SSRIs). In addition, research has proven that an acute, temporary relapse of depressive signs may be produced in studies topics in remission the use of tryptophan depletion, which reasons a transient discount in CNS five-HT degrees. However, the impact of SSRIs on 5HT reuptake is immediate, however the antidepressant impact calls for publicity of numerous weeks' duration. Also, a few antidepressants don't have any impact on 5HT (e.g., desipramine), and the antidepressant tianeptine complements 5HT uptake. All this, collectively with preclinical studies findings, implies a position for neuronal receptor law, intracellular signaling, and gene expression over the years, similarly to more desirable neurotransmitter availability.

Seasonal affective disease is a shape of foremost depressive disease that normally arises at some point of the autumn and iciness and resolves at some point of the spring and summer. Studies endorse that seasonal affective disease is likewise mediated through changes in CNS degrees of five-HT and looks to be induced through changes in circadian rhythm and daylight publicity.

Vascular lesions might also additionally make contributions to despair through disrupting the neural networks concerned in emotion law—particularly, frontostriatal pathways that hyperlink the dorsolateral prefrontal cortex, orbitofrontal cortex, anterior cingulate, and dorsal cingulate. Other additives of limbic circuitry, particularly the hippocampus and amygdala, were implicated in despair.

Brain systems

Functional neuroimaging research help the speculation that the depressed kingdom is related to reduced metabolic hobby in neocortical systems and multiplied metabolic hobby in limbic systems. Serotonergic neurons implicated in affective issues are located within the dorsal raphe nucleus, the limbic device, and the left prefrontal cortex.

A meta-evaluation evaluating mind systems in sufferers with foremost despair, in wholesome controls, and in sufferers with bipolar disease validated institutions among despair and multiplied lateral ventricle size, large cerebrospinal fluid extent, and smaller volumes of the basal ganglia, thalamus, hippocampus, frontal lobe, orbitofrontal cortex, and gyrus rectus. Patients experiencing a depressive episode had smaller hippocampal extent than the ones in remission.

In one look at, positron emission tomographic (PET) photos confirmed abnormally dwindled hobby in a place of the prefrontal cortex in sufferers with unipolar despair and bipolar despair. This vicinity is associated with emotional reaction and has tremendous connections with different regions of the mind, together with the regions that look like chargeable for the law of DA, noradrenaline (locus ceruleus), and five-HT (raphe nuclei).

Both purposeful and structural abnormalities had been located within the identical mind vicinity at some point of a primary depressive episode. Sacher et al located will increase in glucose metabolism within the proper subgenual and pregenual anterior cingulate cortices and reduced grey be counted volumes withinside the amygdala, dorsal frontomedian cortex, and proper paracingulate cortex.

Aging

An integrative version of past due-onset despair posits that age-associated mind adjustments and sickness-associated adjustments (e.g., cerebrovascular sickness), coupled with physiologic vulnerabilities (e.g., genetic hazard elements, private records of despair) and psychosocial adversity, cause disruptions within the purposeful circuitry of emotion law—namely, hypometabolism of cortical systems and hypermetabolism of limbic systems.

Endocrine adjustments in despair are glaring throughout the existence span, however a few are precise to growing older. Women with a preceding records of despair are at better hazard of growing despair at some point of menopause, even though estrogen substitute does now no longer relieve despair; low testosterone degrees were related to despair in older guys.

Etiology

The precise purpose of foremost depressive disease isn't always recognized. As with maximum psychiatric issues, foremost depressive disease seems to be a multifactorial and heterogeneous institution of issues regarding each genetic and environmental element.

Evidence from own circle of relatives and dual research shows that with despair that develops in early childhood, the transmission from dad and mom to kids seems to be associated extra to psychosocial affects than to genetics. Adolescent-onset and grownup-onset despair, whilst extra heritable than prepubertal despair, likewise replicate an interplay among genes and environmental stressors.

Genetics

Genetic elements play an essential position within the improvement of foremost despair. Evidence from dual research shows that foremost despair has a concordance of 40-50%. First-diploma loved ones of depressed people are approximately three instances as probably to expand despair as the overall populace; however, despair can arise in human beings without own circle of relatives histories of despair, as properly.

Two susceptibility loci were recognized wherein no precise gene of hobby has been definitively recognized. The MDD1 locus is placed at 12q22-q23.2 and is maximum strongly connected to foremost despair in men. The MDD2 locus is placed at 15q25.2-q26.2 and has been related to early onset or recurrent episodes of despair.

Although more than one genes are probably to steer the susceptibility to despair, the ones concerned within the serotonin device are a focal point of investigation, particularly due to the fact many antidepressant medicinal drugs paintings through influencing serotonin. The SLC6A4 gene, that is placed at 17q11.2, encodes a serotonin transporter (additionally called five-hydroxytryptamine transporter) this is chargeable for actively clearing serotonin from the synaptic space.

A polymorphism withinthe promoter vicinity of the SLC6A4 gene includes a 44bp insertion or deletion regarding repeat elements. These polymorphisms are called both an extended allele or a quick allele. Caspi et al located that men and women who had been homozygous or heterozygous for the fast allele had extra depressive signs and suicidality in affiliation with demanding existence occasions than the ones sufferers who had been homozygous for the lengthy allele.

Other research additionally endorses that genes controlling both the manufacturing or usage of serotonin play an essential position within the pathogenesis of despair. The TPH2 gene encodes tryptophan hydroxylase, that is the fee-restricting enzyme within the synthesis of serotonin. An in vitro look at of a TPH2 polymorphism, R441H, located at about 80% loss in serotonin manufacturing.

The medical importance of this polymorphism stays unsure, however. Zhang et al located that the allele became extra not unusualplace in a cohort of sufferers with foremost despair than in a manage populace, however a later look at through Garriock et al did now no longer discover any sufferers with the R441H mutation in a cohort with foremost despair, a manage institution, or a collection with bipolar disease.

The HTR3A and HTR3B regions, which encode serotonin receptors and are positioned at chromosome 11q23.2, also are regarded to be related to predominant despair in each European and Japanese populations. Yamada e al surveyed 29 polymorphisms positioned in the HTR3A and HTR3B genes and located a unmarried-nucleotide polymorphism that turned into related to despair in women.

A have a look at of genes within the hypothalamic-pituitary-adrenal axis located that during sufferers with predominant despair, homozygosity for the T allele within the FKBP5 gene turned into related to a faster reaction to antidepressants than heterozygosity or homozygosity for the C allele in that location. However, homozygosity for the T allele turned into additionally related to a multiplied recurrence of depressive episodes.

Studies consisting of the ones suggested with the aid of using Akiskal and Weller and Weissman et al propose a genetic element within the etiology of depressive issues. Individuals with an own circle of relatives records of affective issues, panic sickness, or alcohol dependence bring a better chance for predominant depressive sickness.

Children and youth

Nobile et al located that human platelet five-HT uptake is differentially motivated in kids and youth with and without despair with the aid of using a not unusualplace genetic variation of the promoter location of the serotonin transporter gene (five-HTTLPR). Depressed people had a decrease fee of serotonin uptake and a decrease serotonin dissociation regular

Birmaher et al located that earlier than the onset of affective infection, kids who had been at excessive chance for despair, on the premise of own circle of relatives records, had the identical sample of neuroendocrine reaction to infusion of a serotonergic precursor (five-hydroxy-L-tryptophan) task as did kids with predominant despair. Compared with low-chance kids, excessive-chance kids and depressed kids secreted notably much less cortisol and, in women, greater prolactin. These findings ought to represent the identity of a trait marker for despair in kids.

Late-onset despair

Some proof shows that past due-onset despair (after age 60 years) is an etiologically and clinically wonderful syndrome and that genetic elements possibly play much less of a function in past due-onset despair than in early-onset despair. An own circle of relatives records of despair is much less not unusualplace amongst sufferers with past due-onset despair than in more youthful adults with despair. However, despite the fact that findings were inconsistent, positive genetic markers were located to be related to past due-onset despair. Such markers consist of polymorphisms of apolipoprotein E, BDNF, and five-HT transporter genes. Interestingly, those markers have additionally been related to cognitive impairment, hippocampal volume, and antidepressant reaction, respectively.

Genetic effects on antidepressant drug reaction

Genetics additionally play a widespread component within the reaction to pharmacologic remedy of predominant despair. A have a look at of the drug transporter gene ABCB1 (which encodes a transporter glycoprotein and features as a lively efflux pump for some of tablets throughout the blood-mind barrier) located an affiliation among 2 unmarried-nucleotide polymorphisms and success of remission with citalopram, paroxetine, amitriptyline, and venlafaxine. Also, in a mouse version missing the gene homologous to the human ABCB1 gene, the mice had notably better concentrations of citalopram, venlafaxine, or desvenlafaxine after eleven days of subcutaneous management of the tablets, regardless of drug plasma concentrations that had been same to the ones in mice missing this mutation.

Approximately 40% of sufferers who're dealt with a selective serotonin reuptake inhibitor (SSRI) will both stop remedy or transfer medicines due to an unfavorable impact of the medicinal drug. In one have a look at, an multiplied chance for sexual disorder from SSRIs turned into located to be related to alleles within the 5HT2A and GHB3 genes

A have a look at of reaction to remedy with citalopram recognized a widespread affiliation among remedy final results and a marker in HTR2A, that is positioned at chromosome 13q14.2 and encodes the serotonin 2A receptor. The A allele (an unmarried-nucleotide polymorphism in an intron of this gene) decreased the probability of nonresponse to citalopram in whites however now no longer within the African-American populace. An AA genotype ended in a 16-18% discount in absolute chance of being a nonresponder.

Stressors

Although predominant depressive sickness can rise up with none precipitating stressors, strain and interpersonal losses simply boom chance. For example, lack of a determine earlier than the age of 10 years will increase the chance of later despair. Cognitive-behavioral fashions of despair posit that poor cognitions and underlying all-or-not anything schemata make a contribution to and perpetuate depressed temper.

Chronic ache, scientific infection, and psychosocial strain also can play a function in predominant depressive sickness. Older adults can also additionally locate scientific infection psychologically distressing, and those ailments can also additionally result in multiplied incapacity, reduced independence, and disruption of social networks. Chronic aversive signs consisting of ache related to persistent scientific infection can also additionally disrupt sleep and different biorhythms main to despair.

Other psychosocial chance elements for despair in past due lifestyles consist of the subsequent:

- Impaired social supports
- Caregiver burden
- Loneliness
- Bereavement

Negative lifestyles occasions

Cognitive-behavioral fashions of despair propose that the presence of poor lifestyles occasions similarly to one's notion of or response to the ones occasions can also additionally effect the improvement and protection of depressive signs. Cognitive fashions of despair posit that poor cognitions and underlying all-or-not anything schemata make a contribution to and perpetuate depressed temper. More particularly, cognitive vulnerability-strain fashions propose that, within the face of poor lifestyles occasions, people who've a bent to make poor attributions approximately the reasons of these occasions, approximately themselves, and approximately destiny consequences (in step with the hopelessness concept of despair) can be much more likely to broaden despair. This has been cautioned as probably contributing to gender variations in charges of despair following puberty (e.g., Hyde, Mezulis, and Abramson [35]). Behavioral fashions propose that despair can also additionally end result from deficits in reaction-contingent advantageous reinforcement and inadequate social skills or reliance upon break out and avoidance behaviors, such that avoidance behaviors in reaction to poor lifestyles occasions and corresponding poor feelings can also additionally result in worsened despair.

In addition, neurochemical hypotheses factor to the deleterious consequences of cortisol and different strain-associated materials at the neuronal substrate of temper within the CNS.

Exposure to positive pharmacologic dealers will increase the chance of despair, consisting of reserpine, beta-blockers, and steroids consisting of cortisol. Abused materials also can boom chance of predominant depressive sickness, consisting of cocaine, amphetamine, narcotics, and alcohol. With dealers of abuse, however, it's far uncertain whether or not despair is an outcome or facilitator.

Risk-aspect interactions

Researchers are presently investigating the connection among genetic vulnerability, environmental stressors, and mind structural abnormalities within the improvement of despair. In an MRI genetic have a look at, Frodl et al located that sufferers with predominant despair who carried the S allele of five-HTTLPR and had a records of adolescence emotional overlook had smaller hippocampal volumes than sufferers who had best one of these elements. They concluded that structural hippocampal mind modifications as a consequence of strain can be a part of the chance for growing despair and that those modifications are greater stated in people with the S-allele.

Conflicting proof exists concerning the interplay among the practical serotonin transporter promoter (five-HTTLPR) and strain within the improvement of despair. A 2011 meta-evaluation cautioned that five-HTTLPR moderates the connection among strain and despair. Earlier, smaller meta-analyses had concluded that the proof did now no longer help the presence of the interplay.

Neuroendocrine abnormalities and neurodegenerative diseases

Possible abnormalities of the neurotransmitter structures stay beneath investigation. Compared with manipulate subjects, depressed prepubertal kids had decrease cortisol secretion throughout the primary four hours of sleep, in step with De Bellis et al. Nocturnal secretion of adrenocorticotropic, boom hormone, and prolactin did now no longer vary among the two groups.

Potential organic chance elements were recognized for despair within the aged. Neurodegenerative diseases (particularly Alzheimer disease and Parkinson disease), stroke, a couple of sclerosis, seizure issues, cancer, macular degeneration, and persistent ache were related to better charges of despair. Alternatively, a massive, longitudinal have a look at located that despair that begins offevolved early in lifestyles will increase the chance for Alzheimer's ailment (AD). Researchers used facts from the Prospective Population Study of Women in Gothenburg Sweden, which started in 1968. The have a look at pattern blanketed 800 ladies (imply age, forty-six years), born among 1914 and 1930, who had been observed up with in 1974, 1980, 1992, 2000, 2009, and 2012. Data display the ones ladies who skilled the onset of despair earlier than age twenty years had been 3 instances much more likely to broaden AD (adjusted HR, three.41; 95% CI, 1.78 - 6.54).

Parent-toddler relations

The determine-toddler relation version conceptualizes despair because the end result of terrible determine-toddler interplay. Adults with despair document low paternal involvement and excessive maternal overprotection throughout early adolescence. Troubled relationships with dad and mom, siblings, and friends are not unusualplace in kids and youth with affective infection.

Affective infection in a determine can be a aspect in toddler abuse and/or overlook that promotes affective infection within the toddler. Childhood abuse and overlook, in addition to a cumulative load of stressors over a lifetime, were related to each early-person and past due-onset despair.

Hammen et al suggested a widespread temporal affiliation among despair diagnoses in mom and toddler. They located that kids with vast strain publicity who additionally had symptomatic moms had been notably greater depressed than kids who had been uncovered to similar degrees of strain best.

Mothers' remission from despair, irrespective of timing, has a continually favorable have an impact on their kids. In the Sequenced Treatment Alternatives to Relieve Depression (STAR*D) Child have a look at, all kids whose moms skilled remission from despair confirmed development in temper and conduct within the following 12 months; kids whose moms recovered from despair in the first three months of remedy confirmed now no longer best advanced temper and conduct however widespread development in functioning, as well.

Vascular despair

The vascular despair speculation posits that cerebrovascular ailment can also additionally reason or make a contribution to past due-lifestyles despair. Various traces of proof help this speculation, inclusive of the subsequent:

- Higher prevalence of despair following a left-sided stroke
- Higher occurrence of ischemic white-be counted modifications in older adults with despair than the ones with out
- Bidirectional affiliation among despair and coronary artery ailment and despair and diabetes

- Higher charges of despair amongst sufferers with vasculardementia than people with Alzheimer ailment

Epidemiology

United States information

According to the CDC, in 2019, 2.8% of adults skilled excessive signs of despair, four.2% skilled mild signs, and 11.5% skilled slight signs within the beyond 2 weeks. The percent of adults who skilled any signs of despair turned into maximum amongst the ones elderly 18–29 years (21.0%), observed with the aid of using the ones elderly 45–sixty four years (18.4%) and sixty five and older (18.4%), and lastly, with the aid of using the ones elderly 30–forty four years (16.8%). Women had been much more likely than guys to enjoy slight, mild, or excessive signs of despair. Non-Hispanic Asian adults had been least possibly to enjoy slight, mild, or excessive signs of despair as compared with Hispanic, non-Hispanic white, and non-Hispanic black adults.

International information

Internationally suggested person occurrence charges of despair typically replicate the ones of the United States, and estimates of 1-month occurrence of despair in community-residing aged are fairly steady (e.g., England, 2.9%; The Netherlands, 2.0%; Sweden, 5.6%; Nigeria, 1.6%). However, sparse facts are to be had at the worldwide prevalence of predominant despair in kids and youth.

Helgason tested the complete Icelandic beginning cohort of 1895-ninety-seven with periodic follow-up till cohort people reached age 74–seventy-six years. The lifetime estimates of chance for any affective sickness had been 14.8% for women and nine.8% for adult males. The World Health Organization(WHO) collaborative have a look at the evaluation of depressive issues located extensive similarity in depressive symptomatology throughout cultures in Canada, Iran, Japan, and Switzerland.

The Stirling County Study, which started rapidly after World War II, supplied a 40-12 months' angle of the superiority and prevalence of psychiatric issues in a person populace in Atlantic Canada, wherein the general occurrence of despair remained strong at five◆ross three separate samples in 1952, 1970, and 1992. In the 2000 pattern, however, the superiority had shifted from older to more youthful people, and the lady-to-male ratio had multiplied.

Copeland et al located extensively ranging prevalences for despair in aged people in nine European populations. The occurrence for women turned into better than that for adult males, and there has been no regular affiliation among occurrence and age. Meta-evaluation found out a universal occurrence of 12.3% and frequencies of 14.1% for women and 8.6% for adult males.

Children and youth

According to the CDC, in 2016–2019, 4.4% (2.7 million) kids elderly three–17 years had been recognized with despair.

The prevalence of despair turned into 0.9% in preschool-elderly kids, 1.9% in college-elderly kids, and 4.7% in youth in a have a look at with the aid of using Kashani and Sherman. In some other have a look at, greater than 22% of lady excessive college students and greater than eleven% of male excessive college students suggested 1 contemporary or lifetime episode of unipolar despair. The percent of male college students with 2 or greater episodes of unipolar despair turned into 4.9%; it turned into 1.6% in lady college students.

In prepubertal kids, boys and women are affected equally. Hankin et al located that the maximum vital time for intercourse variations in despair to emerge is from age 15–18 years. During this duration, the boom in universal charges of despair and onset of latest instances of despair top.

Hispanic youths in Los Angeles county (elderly 12–17 years) suggested greater signs of despair, impartial of socioeconomic repute, while as compared with white, black, or Asian American youth, the use of the Children's Depression Inventory (CDI). This have a look at additionally located widespread consequences of social elegance on despair. As earnings reduced, the common occurrence of despair multiplied.

Elderly people

Although charges of despair in men and women are maximum in the ones elderly 25–forty-four years, the prevalence of clinically widespread depressive signs will increase with advancing age, particularly while related to scientific infection or institutionalization. However, the despair may not meet standards for predominant despair due to quite ordinary capabilities of despair in aged people. For instance, there may be a better occurrence of dysthymic sickness in growing old and medically sick populations.

Prognosis

Major depressive sickness has widespread capacity morbidity and mortality, contributing because it does to suicide, prevalence and unfavorable consequences of scientific infection, disruption in interpersonal relationships, substance abuse, and misplaced paintings time. With suitable remedy, 70-80% of people with predominant depressive sickness can attain a widespread discount in signs, despite the fact that as many as 50% of sufferers might not reply to the preliminary remedy trial.

Twenty percentage of people with predominant depressive sickness untreated at 1 12 months will keep to satisfy standards for the analysis, while a further 40% may have a partial remission. Pretreatment irritability and psychotic signs can be related to poorer consequences. Partial remission and/or a records of earlier persistent predominant depressive episodes are chance elements for recurrent episodes and remedy resistance.

A have a look at of first-episode psychotic despair with the aid of using Tohen et al located that maximum sufferers finished syndromal remission (86%) and healing (84%); however, best 35% recovered functionally. Earlier syndromal healing turned into related to subacute onset, decrease preliminary despair ratings, and shortage of temper-incongruent psychotic capabilities. Within 2 years, nearly 1/2 of the sufferers skilled new episodes. In 41% of sufferers, the analysis turned into changed, normally to bipolar or schizoaffective issues.

Recurrence of early despair

According to the American Academy of Child and Adolescent Psychiatry(AACAP) exercise parameters for depressive issues in adolescence and adolescence, a records of a preceding depressive episode, subsyndromal signs of despair, dysthymia, and tension issues boom the chance for destiny despair. In a have a look at of an epidemiologic pattern of 776 youth with the aid of using Pine and associates, signs of major depression in adolescence strongly anticipated episodes of predominant despair in adulthood.

Late-onset despair

The diagnosis for sufferers with past due-onset despair is felt to be poorer than that for more youthful sufferers, and it seems to be depending on bodily incapacity or infection and shortage of social help. Of precise significance is the growing chance of demise with the aid of using suicide, mainly amongst aged guys. The duration of a depressive episode within the growing old populace is about 18 months, while in humans 20–fifty five years of age, the duration of an episode is eighteen to 24 weeks.

In older sufferers, despair is regularly comorbid with persistent scientific situations and may result in worsening scientific consequences, inclusive of mortality. For example, coronary artery ailment is a chance aspect for the improvement of despair, and despair is an impartial chance aspect for the improvement of coronary ailment. Patients with each situation are much more likely to die than people with coronary artery ailment alone. Both behavioral and physiologic motives are possibly for those associations.

Millard cautioned the "rule of thirds" regarding the diagnosis of past due-onset despair, which states that irrespective of remedy, about one 1/3 of sufferers will happen remission, some other one 1/3 will stay symptomatic within the identical condition, and the final one 1/3 will worsen. In reality, studies have proven that about 60% of sufferers with past due-onset despair may have at the least 1 recurrence, and as much as 40% of those sufferers may have persistent or constantly recurrent despair.

Late-onset despair has been suggested to double the chance of growing mild cognitive impairment and the probability that the slight impairment will grow to be dementia. The Diabetes and Aging Study confirmed that once despair is comorbid with kind 2 diabetes, it will increase the chance of all-reason dementia with the aid of using approximately 2-fold as compared with diabetes alone. A 40-month have a look at of 2977 middle-elderly and older adults with lengthy-status kind 2 diabetes located despair at baseline to be related to elevated cognitive decline.

Compared with contributors without a despair records, people with past due-lifestyles despair reportedly have multiplied all-reason dementia chance; however, early-lifestyles despair had no affiliation with dementia chance. Treating despair has been cautioned to probable stunt development to slight cognitive impairment after which to dementia, despite the fact that there was little assessment of this speculation to date.

Suicide

Depression performs a function in multiple 1/2 of all suicide tries, while the lifetime chance of suicide amongst sufferers with untreated depressive sickness is almost 20%. According to Centers for Disease Control and Prevention (CDC) facts, suicide charges multiplied 30�tween 2000 and 2018, and declined in 2019 and 2020. Suicide is a main reason of demise within the United States, with 45,979 deaths in 2020. This is ready one demise each eleven minutes. The wide variety of folks who consider or strive suicide is even better. In 2020, an envisioned 12.2 million American adults significantly notion approximately suicide, 3.2 million deliberate a suicide strive, and 1.2 million tried suicide.

Suicide impacts all a long time. In 2020, suicide turned into most of the pinnacle nine main reasons of demise for humans a long time 10–sixty-four. Suicide turned into the second one main reason of demise for humans a long time 10–14 and 25–34.

However, regardless of those facts and the reality that despair is greater regularly recognized in ladies, the best suicide fee is in guys older than seventy-five years; greater guys than ladies die from suicide with the aid of using an aspect of 4.5:1. White guys whole greater than 78% of all suicides, and 56% of suicide deaths in adult males contain firearms. Poisoning is the fundamental approach amongst women. Attempted suicide is greater common in ladies.

- Diagnosis of predominant despair
- Previous records of suicide tries
- Depressive signs with agitation or misery

Burden of scientific ailment and the presence of a contemporary extreme scientific condition (despite the fact that this chance can be mediated with the aid of using an analysis of despair)

Recent annoying lifestyles occasions, particularly own circle of relative's discord

- Lack of social help
- Being widowed or divorced
- The presence of a gun within the home
- Unexplained weight reduction
- High degrees of tension
- Lack of a cause now no longer to devote suicide

- Presence of a selected plan that may be carried out
- Rehearsal of the plan

The dating among use of antidepressants and chance of suicide varies with affected person age. Treatment with antidepressants has been related to multiplied suicidality in kids, youth, and teens 18 to 24 years of age. There isn't any proof of multiplied chance for adults older than 24 years of age; for adults sixty-five years of age or older, the chance is simply reduced.

Suicide charges amongst Native Americans and Alaskan Natives among a long time 15 and 34 years are nearly two times the countrywide common for this age variety. Hispanic women make notably greater suicide tries than their male or non-Hispanic counterparts.

In one have a look at, there had been robust correlations of suicide charges with signs of get entry to fitness care within the United States. Multivariate evaluation of kingdom-with the aid of using-kingdom information confirmed that the kingdom fee of federal useful resource for intellectual fitness turned into the most powerful indicator, observed with the aid of using the fee of uninsured people and populace density of psychiatrists and physicians and with the aid of using populace density. These researchers concluded that the findings help the view that scientific intervention is an important detail within the prevention of suicide.

More than 77% of world suicides befell in low- and middle-earnings nations in 2019. It is envisioned that round 20% of world suicides are because of pesticide self-poisoning, maximum of which arise in rural agricultural regions in low- and middle-earnings nations. Other not unsualplace techniques of suicide are putting and firearms.

Patient Education

Education performs a critical function within a hit remedy of predominant depressive sickness. Over the lengthy time period, sufferers may additionally turn out to be aware about symptoms and symptoms of relapse and can are seeking for remedy early. Patients need to be aware about the intent in the back of the selection of remedy, capacity unfavorable consequences, and anticipated effects. The involvement of the affected person within the remedy plan can beautify medicinal drug compliance and referral to counseling.

Family contributors additionally want training approximately the character of despair and can gain from supportive interactions. Engaging own circle of relatives may be a vital element of a remedy plan, particularly for pediatric and past due-onset despair. Family contributors are beneficial informants, can make sure medicinal drug compliance, and may inspire sufferers to alternate behaviors that perpetuate despair (e.g., inactivity).

The following net web sites are treasured sources for affected person and own circle of relatives training:

- National Institute of Mental Health: Depression
- MedlinePlus: Depression
- FamilyDoctor.org: Depression
- DepressionandBipolarSupportAlliance(DBSA)
- FamiliesforDepressionAwareness

Helpful net web sites particularly for past due-onset despair consist of the subsequent:

- MedlinePlus: Depression-aged
- National Institute of Mental Health: Older Adults: Depression and Suicide Facts
- University of Maryland Medical Center: Depression-aged

Depression Clinical Presentation

History

Patients with predominant depressive sickness might not first of all gift with a grievance of low temper, anhedonia, or different traditional signs. In the number one care putting, in which lots of those sufferers first are seeking for remedy, the offering court cases regularly may be somatic (e.g., fatigue, headache, belly misery, or alternate in weight). Patients can also additionally whinge greater of irritability or trouble concentrating than of unhappiness or low temper.

Children with predominant depressive sickness may additionally gift with first of all deceptive signs consisting of irritability, decline in college performance, or social withdrawal. Elderly people can also additionally gift with confusion or a standard decline in functioning; additionally, they enjoy greater somatic court cases, cognitive signs, and less court cases of unhappy or dysphoric temper.

Familial, social, and environmental elements

Depression may be familial. Thus, a radical own circle of relatives records is pretty critical. Familial, social, and environmental elements seem to play widespread roles within the path of depressive infection in kids and youths, even in preschool kids. René Spitz defined anaclitic despair (marasmus) in babies being raised in an orphanage and in hospitalized kids whose dad and mom had been now no longer allowed to visit.

Dysphoric temper

A dysphoric temper kingdom can be expressed with the aid of using sufferers as unhappiness, heaviness, numbness, or now and again irritability and temper swings. They regularly document a lack of hobby or satisfaction of their regular sports, trouble concentrating, or lack of power and motivation. Their wondering is regularly poor, regularly with emotions of worthlessness, hopelessness, or helplessness.

Psychosis

Patients with predominant depressive sickness typically display ruminative wondering. Nevertheless, it's far critical to assess every affected person for proof of psychotic signs, due to the fact this impacts preliminary management.

Psychosis, while it happens within the context of unipolar despair, is normally congruent in its content material with the affected person's temper kingdom; for example, the affected person can also additionally enjoy delusions of worthlessness or a few innovative bodily decline.

Symptoms of psychosis need to activate a cautious records assessment to rule out any of the subsequent:

- Bipolar affective sickness
- Schizophrenia
- Schizoaffective sickness
- Substance abuse
- Organic mind syndrome

Physical Examination

No bodily findings are particular to predominant depressive sickness; instead, the analysis is primarily based totally at the records and the intellectual repute exam. Nevertheless, a whole intellectual fitness assessment need to constantly consist of a scientific assessment to rule out natural situations that would imitate a depressive sickness. Most of those fall into the subsequent predominant standard categories:

- Infection
- Medication
- Endocrine sickness
- Tumor
- Neurologic sickness

Appearance and have an effect on

Most sufferers with predominant depressive sickness gift with an ordinary appearance. In sufferers with greater excessive signs, a decline in grooming and hygiene may be found, in addition to an alternate in weight. Patients can also additionally display psychomotor retardation, which manifests as a slowing or lack of spontaneous motion and reactivity, in addition to display a knocking down or lack of reactivity within the affected persons have an effect on (i.e., emotional expression). Psychomotor agitation or restlessness also can be found in a few sufferers with predominant depressive sickness.

Speech

Speech can be ordinary, slow, monotonic, or missing in spontaneity and content material. Pressured speech need to propose tension or mania, while disorganized speech need to activate an assessment for psychosis. Racing mind can also be a demonstration of tension, mania, or hypomania.

Major Depressive Disorder

The particular DSM-five standards for predominant depressive sickness are mentioned below.

At least five of the subsequent signs should were gift throughout the identical 2-week duration (and at the least 1 of the signs should be faded hobby/satisfaction or depressed temper):

- Depressed temper: For kids and youth, this could additionally be an irritable temper
- Diminished hobby or lack of satisfaction in nearly all sports (anhedonia)
- Significant weight alternate or urge for food disturbance: For kids, this could be failure to attain anticipated weight gain
- Sleep disturbance (insomnia or hypersomnia)
- Psychomotor agitation or retardation
- Fatigue or lack of power
- Feelings of worthlessness

- Diminished cappotential to assume or concentrate; indecisiveness
- Recurrent mind of demise, recurrent suicidal ideation without a selected plan, or a suicide strive or particular plan for committing suicide

The signs reason widespread misery or impairment in social, occupational or different critical regions of functioning.

The signs aren't as a consequence of the physiological consequences of a substance (e.g., a drug of abuse, a medicinal drug) or some other scientific condition.

The disturbance isn't always higher defined with the aid of using a chronic schizoaffective sickness, schizophrenia, delusional sickness, or different particular or unspecified schizophrenia spectrum and different psychotic issues

There has in no way been a manic episode or a hypomanic episode

Depressive issues may be rated as slight, mild, or excessive. The sickness also can arise with psychotic signs, which may be temper congruent or incongruent. Depressive issues may be decided to be in complete or partial remission.

DSM-five similarly notes the significance of distinguishing among ordinary unhappiness and grief from a first-rate depressive sickness. While bereavement can set off super suffering, it does now no longer commonly set off a first-rate depressive sickness. When the 2 exist concurrently, the signs and practical impairment is greater excessive and the diagnosis is worse as compared to bereavement alone. When predominant depressive sickness is maximum possibly to be precipitated with the aid of using bereavement in people with different vulnerabilities to depressive issues. An analysis of predominant depressive sickness following a widespread loss calls for scientific judgement primarily based totally at the people records and the cultural context for expression of grief.

Depression with Anxious Distress

Anxious misery is described because the presence of at the least 2 of the subsequent signs:

- Feeling keyed up or tense

- Feeling strangely restless
- Difficulty concentrating due to worry
- Fear that something lousy can also additionally happen
- Feeling of capacity lack of manipulate

Severity is similarly particular as:

- Mild: Two signs
- Moderate: Three signs
- Moderate-excessive: Four or 5 signs
- Severe: Four or 5 signs with motor agitation

High degrees of tension are related to better suicide chance, longer length of infection and more probability of nonresponse to remedy.

Depression with Melancholic Features

In despair with melancholic capabilities, both a lack of satisfaction in nearly all sports or a loss of reactivity to normally fulfilling stimuli is gift. Additionally, at the least three of the subsequent are required:

- A depressed temper this is tremendously one of a kind from the sort this is felt while a cherished one is deceased
- Depression this is worse within the morning
- Waking up 2 hours in advance than regular
- Observable psychomotor retardation or agitation
- Significant weight reduction or anorexia
- Excessive or irrelevant guilt

According to DSM-five, this subtype is implemented best while there may be a near-whole absence of the ability for satisfaction, now no longer simply a diminution. A depressed temper this is defined as simply greater excessive, longer lasting or gift without a cause isn't always taken into consideration a wonderful quality. Melancholic capabilities are greater common in inpatients and are much less possibly to arise in milder predominant depressive episodes.

They also are much more likely to be comorbid with psychotic capabilities.

Depression with Catatonia

The DSM-five standards for analysis of depressive episodes with catatonia calls for the presence of three or greater of 12 psychomotor capabilities throughout maximum of the episode:

- Stupor
- Catalepsy
- Waxy flexibility
- Mutism
- Negativism
- Posturing
- Mannerism
- Stereotypy
- Agitation, now no longer motivated with the aid of using outside stimuli
- Grimacing
- Echolalia
- Echopraxia

Atypical Depression

An episode of despair can be recognized as having ordinary capabilities. Characteristics of this subtype are temper reactivity and exclusion of melancholic and catatonic subtypes similarly to two or greater of the subsequent for a duration of at the least 2 weeks:

- Increased urge for food or widespread weight gain
- Increased sleep

Feelings of heaviness in fingers or sensitivities of the legs that make bigger a way past the temper disturbance episodes and bring about widespread impairment in social or occupational functioning

A sample of longstanding interpersonal rejection sensitivity that extends a way past the temper disturbance episodes and effects in widespread impairment in social or occupational functioning.

Postpartum Depression

Depression within the postpartum duration is a not unusualplace and probably very extreme problem; as much as 85% of ladies can broaden temper disturbances throughout this duration. For maximum ladies, signs are temporary and comparatively slight (i.e., "postpartum blues"); however, 10-15% of ladies enjoy a greater disabling and chronic shape of depression, with an onset later than the postpartum blues, and 0.1-0.2% of ladies enjoy postpartum psychosis.

Postpartum psychiatric infection turned into first of all conceptualized as a collection of issues particularly connected to being pregnant and childbirth and accordingly turned into taken into consideration diagnostically wonderful from different sorts of psychiatric infection. However, proof in the beyond decade shows that postpartum psychiatric infection is truly indistinguishable from psychiatric issues that arise at different instances throughout a woman's lifestyles. However, the probability of a bipolar final results is significantly better in postpartum psychosis.

Postpartum temper sickness (predominant depressive or manic) episodes with psychotic capabilities seem to arise in from 1 in 500 to one in one thousand deliveries. The chance is mainly multiplied for ladies with earlier postpartum temper episodes however is likewise extended for people with a previous record of a depressive or bipolar sickness or a own circle of relatives records of bipolar sickness. Women who've had a postpartum episode with psychotic capabilities have a chance of recurrence among 30-50% for next deliveries.

Rapidly fluctuating temper, tearfulness, irritability, and tension are not unusualplace signs of postpartum blues. Symptoms top at the fourth or 5th day after shipping and closing for numerous days, however they're typically time-restrained and spontaneously remit in the first 2 postpartum weeks. Symptoms do now no longer intrude with a mom's cappotential to feature and to take care of her toddler.

Women with greater excessive signs or signs persisting longer than 2 weeks need to be screened for postpartum despair. According to DSM-five, 50% of "postpartum" predominant depressive episodes simply start previous to shipping, and the specifier used together for those episodes is "with peripartum onset."

Signs and signs of postpartum despair are clinically indistinguishable from predominant despair that happens in ladies at different instances. These signs intrude with the mom's cappotential to feature, with chance of self-damage or damage to the toddler.

The American Academy of Pediatrics (AAP) states that greater than 400,000 babies are born every 12 months to moms who're depressed. The AAP encourages pediatric practices to create a device to higher perceive postpartum despair to make sure a more healthy determine-toddler dating.

Although powerful nonpharmacologic and pharmacologic remedies are to be had, each sufferers and their caregivers regularly forget postpartum despair. Untreated postpartum affective infection locations each the mom and toddler at chance and is related to widespread lengthy-time period consequences on toddler improvement and conduct; therefore, suitable screening, activate recognition, and remedy of despair are critical for each maternal and toddler wellbeing and may enhance consequences.

Seasonal Affective Disorder

About 70% of depressed humans sense worse throughout the wintry weather and higher throughout the summer. To meet the DSM-five diagnostic standards for predominant depressive sickness with seasonal sample, despair need to be gift best at a selected time of 12 months (e.g., within the fall or wintry weather) and complete remission happens at a feature time of 12 months (e.g., spring). A character need to display at the least 2 episodes of depressive disturbance within the preceding 2 years, and seasonal episodes need to significantly outnumber nonseasonal episodes. Patients with seasonal affective sickness are much more likely to document ordinary signs, consisting of hypersomnia, multiplied urge for food, and a yearning for carbohydrates.

Cases in which there may be an apparent impact of seasonally associated psychosocial stressors, (e.g., seasonal unemployment) do now no longer meet the diagnostic standards.

Diagnosing seasonal affective sickness in kids is hard due to the fact they enjoy the recurrent widely widespread stressor of starting college each autumn. Also, a younger toddler would possibly gift with obvious seasonal affective sickness however now no longer but have had preceding episodes.

Major Depressive Disorder with Psychotic Features

The presentation of excessive predominant depressive sickness can also additionally consist of psychotic capabilities. Psychotic capabilities consist of delusions and hallucination and can be temper congruent or temper incongruent. Mood-congruent psychoses are regularly steady with conventional depressive issues, consisting of non-public inadequacy, guilt, ailment, or deserved punishment. Mood-incongruent psychoses aren't steady with those traditional issues however may additionally arise in despair.

Major depressive sickness with psychotic capabilities is taken into consideration a psychiatric emergency. Patients can also additionally require psychiatric hospitalization.

Other Specified Depressive Disorders

The DSM-five consists of a class of issues with capabilities of despair that don't meet standards for a selected depressive sickness. Examples consist of the subsequent:

- Recurrent quick despair
- Short length depressive episode

- Depressive episode with inadequate signs

Metabolic Depression

Several research document an affiliation among metabolic syndrome and despair. Vogelzangs et al propose that later in lifestyles, waist circumference and now no longer metabolic syndrome can be expecting onset of despair. Specifically, the bigger the waistline, the better the prevalence of despair. However, longitudinal research has additionally proven that despair predicts next weight problems and centripetal weight problems, possibly due to terrible diet, loss of exercise, and psychobiologic modifications consisting of multiplied cortisol degrees.

On the alternative hand, people with despair who've metabolic syndrome can also additionally in reality be much more likely to have chronic or recurrent despair. Thus, despair with metabolic abnormalities will be classified metabolic despair, a probable persistent subtype of despair.

Cultural Influences on Expression of Depression

Cultural affects at the presentation of despair may be widespread. The practitioner need to be aware about variations within the expression of mental misery in sufferers from different nations or cultures.

Culturally distinct experiences (e.g., worry of being hexed or bewitched; enjoy of visitations from the dead) need to be outstanding from real hallucinations or delusions that can be a part of a first-rate depressive episode with psychotic capabilities.

Suicidal Ideation

Patients with despair need to be assessed for suicidal ideation, particularly if agitation is gift. When an affected person has pondered or tried suicide, the weight is at the fitness care company to at once discover the scenario with the affected person in as a great deal element as feasible to decide the contemporary presence of suicidal ideation in addition to available approach and plans. Discussing those is the maximum critical step clinicians can soak up a try and save you suicide in an at-chance affected person.

Depression Differential Diagnoses

Diagnostic Considerations

The differential analysis for despair consists of an extensive kind of scientific issues, consisting of the subsequent:

- Central worried device diseases (e.g., Parkinson ailment, dementia, a couple of sclerosis, neoplastic lesions)
- Endocrine issues (e.g., hyperthyroidism, hypothyroidism)
- Drug-associated situations (e.g., cocaine abuse, facet consequences of a few CNS depressants)
- Infectious ailment (e.g., mononucleosis)
- Sleep-associated issues

Related psychiatric issues

Major depressive sickness should be differentiated from dysthymia. Patients with dysthymia gift with low temper for at the least 2 years as a number one symptom; they've inadequate signs to satisfy standards for predominant depressive sickness. However, dysthymia can also additionally predate a depressive episode.

Misdiagnosis of bipolar sickness as recurrent unipolar despair can also additionally arise if the clinician does now no longer perceive the presence of hypomania among depressive episodes. This ends in insufficient remedy and, theoretically, ought to result in a precipitation of a hypomanic, manic, or blended episode.

Patients with tension issues are at better chance for growing comorbid despair. In such sufferers, it's far critical to perceive the tension sickness, due to the fact affected people regularly require particular remedy approaches. Commonly encountered tension issues consist of the subsequent:

- Generalized tension sickness
- Obsessive-compulsive sickness
- Panic sickness
- Phobic issues

Posttraumatic strain sickness

Patients with positive character issues (e.g., borderline character sickness) can also additionally gift with temper modifications as an outstanding symptom. Remember that the presence of a character sickness may be hard to decide within the putting of lively affective signs. Many depressed sufferers who seem labile, demanding, or pathologically based appearance dramatically one of a kind as soon as the depressive episode has been dealt with adequately.

People with ingesting issues even have an excessive fee of comorbid predominant depressive sickness and require particular remedy approaches. These issues consist of bulimia, anorexia nervosa, and ingesting sickness now no longer in any other case particular. A massive percent of people on this closing organization have binge-ingesting sickness.

Central worried device issues

Major depressive sickness does now no longer reason focal neurologic symptoms and symptoms. Such findings need to activate an assessment for different natural syndromes.

A wide variety of physiologic and structural CNS techniques can produce modifications in temper and conduct. Note that predominant depressive sickness can produce measurable cognitive deficits or a worsening of preexisting dementia. This decline in cognitive functioning, which on formal checking out seems to rise up from impaired attention or motivation, is called pseudodementia or as dementia of despair and need to remit with a hit remedy of the depressive episode.

Alzheimer ailment and different degenerative and vascular dementias may be related to affective signs, particularly within the preliminary stages of dementia.

Mood issues also are very outstanding in Parkinson ailment, Huntington ailment, a couple of sclerosis, stroke, and seizure issues. Neoplastic lesions of the CNS can reason modifications in temper and conduct earlier than the onset of focal neurologic symptoms and symptoms.

Endocrine issues

Endocrinologic issues regarding the hypothalamic-pituitary-adrenal axis or thyroid are particularly possibly to provide modifications in temper. These consist of Addison ailment, Cushing syndrome, hyperthyroidism, hypothyroidism, prolactinomas, and hyperparathyroidism. A 2018 have a look at located that approximately 45% of humans with depressive issues and 30% of these with tension additionally have autoimmune thyroiditis (AIT).

Drug-associated issues

Pharmacologic dealers can produce modifications in temper. These materials consist of the subsequent:

- Antihypertensive medicines (particularly reserpine and methyldopa)
- Smoking-cessation aids (e.g., varenicline)
- Steroids
- Sex hormones and medicines that have an effect on intercourse hormones (e.g., estrogen, progesterone, testosterone, gonadotropin-freeing hormone [GnRH] antagonists)
- H2 blockers (e.g., ranitidine, cimetidine)
- Sedatives
- Muscle relaxants
- Appetite suppressants
- Chemotherapy dealers (e.g., vincristine, procarbazine, L-asparaginase, interferon, vinblastine)

Among antihypertensive dealers, beta-blockers have a popularity for being strongly related to despair. Research in this affiliation has been quite contradictory, however shows at maximum a minor function on this regard. For example, an assessment with the aid of using Ko et al located no widespread multiplied chance of depressive signs with beta-blockers, despite the fact that there has been a small however widespread chance of fatigue and sexual disorder.

Risk seems to differ with one of a kind beta-blocker. A have a look at with the aid of using Luijendijk in aged sufferers located that relatively lipid-soluble beta-blockers (commonly propranolol) had been related to depressive signs throughout the primary three months of use. In assessment, pindolol can also additionally boost up or beautify the consequences of antidepressant tablets.

Case reviews have cautioned a probable hyperlink among calcium channel blockers and despair. The foremost situation with those dealers, however, is that they'll reason resistance to antidepressants.

Substance use, abuse, or dependence can reason widespread temper signs. This is particularly actual of alcohol, cocaine, amphetamines, cannabinoids, sedatives/hypnotics, and narcotics. Inhalant abuse need to additionally be taken into consideration, mainly amongst younger male sufferers. Other substance-associated and psychiatric techniques both can gift with temper disturbance because the number one symptom or can arise collectively with predominant depressive sickness.

Infectious and inflammatory diseases

Infectious techniques which could reason temper and conduct modifications consist of Lyme ailment, mononucleosis, human immunodeficiency virus (HIV) encephalopathy, and syphilis. Inflammatory situations consisting of systemic lupus erythematosus (SLE) can produce an extensive variety of neuropsychiatric symptoms and symptoms and signs. The possibly mechanism in those instances is changes withinthe blood-mind barrier and an autoimmune cerebritis.

Sleep issues

Of the numerous sleep issues, obstructive sleep apnea specially can reason widespread scientific and psychiatric signs and is regularly overlooked as an analysis. Patients and, if necessary, their companions need to be interviewed concerning their sleep quality, daylight hours' sleepiness, and snoring. Obstructive sleep apnea is particularly not unusualplace in sufferers with weight problems. Polysomnography can assist make the analysis and manual remedy.

Differential Diagnoses

- Adjustment Disorders
- Anemia
- Chronic Fatigue Syndrome (Myalgic Encephalomyelitis)
- Dissociative Disorders
- Illness Anxiety Disorder (previously Hypochondriasis)
- Hypoglycemia
- Hypopituitarism (Panhypopituitarism)
- Schizoaffective Disorder

- Schizophrenia
- Somatic Symptom Disorders
- Depression Workup

Approach Considerations

Depression screening assessments may be treasured, with the maximum extensively one used being the Patient Health Questionnaire-nine (PHQ-nine). It is critical to apprehend, however, that the effects received from using any despair screening or score scales do now no longer diagnose despair and can be imperfect in any populace, particularly in aged sufferers.

Screening Tests

The U.S. Preventive Services Task Force (USPSTF) recommends screening for despair within the standard person populace, inclusive of older adults and pregnant and postpartum ladies. It is critical to apprehend that the effects received from using any despair score scales are imperfect in any populace, particularly the geriatric populace.

The handiest screening takes a look at is an unmarried query: Are you depressed? A pooled evaluation located that unmarried-query screening had a specificity of ninety-seven% however a universal sensitivity of 32% and, accordingly, could perceive best three of each 10 sufferers with despair in number one care.

The following 2-query take a look at addresses depressed temper and anhedonia:

- During the beyond month, have you ever been afflicted with the aid of using feeling down, depressed, or hopeless?
- During the beyond month, have you ever been afflicted with the aid of using little hobby or satisfaction in doing things?

In a cross-sectional have a look at, those 2 screening questions confirmed a sensitivity of ninety-seven% and a specificity of 67%.

Longer self-document screening contraptions for despair consist of the subsequent:

- **PHQ-nine** – The nine-object despair scale of the Patient Health Questionnaire; every object is scored zero to three, imparting a zero to 27 severity rating
- **Beck Depression Inventory (BDI) or Beck Depression Inventory-II (BDI-II)** – 21-query symptom-score scales
- **BDI for number one care** – A 7-query scale tailored from the BDI
- **Zung Self-Rating Depression Scale** – A 20-object survey
- **Center for Epidemiologic Studies-Depression Scale (CES-D)** – A 20-object tool that permits sufferers to assess their emotions, conduct, and outlook from the preceding week

In assessment to the above self-document scales, the Hamilton Depression Rating Scale (HDRS) is accomplished with the aid of using an educated professional, now no longer the affected person. The HDRS has 17 or 21 items, scored from 0-2 or 0-4; a complete rating of 0-7 is taken into consideration ordinary, whilst ratings of 20 or better suggest fairly excessive despair.

Given that the typically ordinary presentation of despair within the aged populace can task even the maximum skilled clinician, score scales within the aged need to be used and interpreted best within the context of a greater thorough exam for despair.

Patients with predominant depressive sickness regularly whinge of terrible reminiscence or attention. This can be because of the despair itself or to an underlying dementia.

In older sufferers with set up dementia, the Cornell Scale for Depression in Dementia may be used to decide the class and severity of despair. The clinician completes the dimensions on the premise of earlier commentary and interviews with the affected person and the affected person's caregiver.

Laboratory Studies to Rule Out Organic Causes

Depression is a medical diagnosis, primarily based totally at the records and bodily findings. No diagnostic laboratory assessments are to be had to diagnose essential depressive sickness, however centered laboratory research can be beneficial to exclude ability clinical ailments that could gift as essential depressive sickness. These laboratory research may encompass the following:

- Complete blood cell (CBC) count
- Thyroid-stimulating hormone (TSH)
- Vitamin B-12
- Rapid plasma reagin (RPR)
- HIV test

- Electrolytes, along with calcium, phosphate, and magnesium levels
- Blood urea nitrogen (BUN) and creatinine
- Liver feature assessments (LFTs)
- Blood alcohol level
- Blood and urine toxicology screen
- Arterial blood gas (ABG)
- Dexamethasone suppression test (Cushing disease, however additionally wonderful in despair)
- Cosyntropin (ACTH) stimulation test (Addison disease)

Neuroimaging

Neuroimaging can assist make clear the character of the neurologic contamination that could produce psychiatric signs, however those research is high priced and can be of questionable price in sufferers without discrete neurologic deficits. Computed tomography (CT) scanning or magnetic resonance imaging (MRI) of the mind have to be taken into consideration if natural mind syndrome or hypopituitarism is protected within the differential diagnosis.

Positron emission tomography (PET) imaging presents the manner for the observe of receptor binding of positive ligands and the impact a compound can also additionally have on receptors. However, PET scanning is elaborate to be used with kids and teenagers as it calls for complicated device and makes use of radiation.

Using unmarried-photon emission computed tomography (SPECT) scanning, Tutus et al stated tremendous variations among the perfusion index values of untreated teenagers with despair and people of manage sufferers. The researchers located that teenagers with essential depressive sickness can also additionally have local blood float deficits within the left anterofrontal and left temporal cortical regions, with extra right-left perfusion asymmetry than wholesome manage sufferers.

Depression Treatment & Management

Approach Considerations

A huge variety of powerful remedies is to be had for essential depressive sickness. Medication on my own (see Medication) and short psychotherapy (e.g., cognitive-behavioral remedy, interpersonal remedy) on my own can relieve depressive signs. There is likewise empirical assist for the capacity of short psychotherapy (CBT) to save you relapse.

In kids and teenagers, however, pharmacotherapy via way of means of itself is inadequate remedy. Moreover, in all affected person populations, the aggregate of drugs and psychotherapy commonly presents the fastest and maximum sustained reaction. Combination remedy has additionally been related to drastically better quotes of development in depressive signs; improved best of life; and higher remedy compliance, specially whilst remedy is wanted for longer than three months.

Medications

Usually, 2–12 weeks at a healing dose, with assumed adherence to the regimen, are wished for a medical reaction to come to be evident. The desire of drugs has to be guided via way of means of predicted protection and tolerability, which useful resource in compliance; medical doctor familiarity, which aids in affected person schooling and anticipation of damaging consequences; and records of preceding remedies. Often, remedy screw ups are because of medicine noncompliance, insufficient length of remedy, or insufficient dosing.

According to the 2008 American College of Physicians (ACP) guiding principle (the maximum latest launch of the guiding principle) on the usage of second-era antidepressants to deal with depressive disorders, affected person alternatives have to receive critical attention whilst deciding on the pleasant direction of pharmacotherapy for sufferers with depressive disorders. The affected person can also additionally need to keep away from use of a selected antidepressant if she or he had a preceding poor revel in with the drug.

The 2008 ACP guiding principle advises that remedy for essential depressive sickness have to be altered if the affected person does now no longer have a good enough reaction to pharmacotherapy inside 6–eight weeks. Once quality reaction is achieved, remedy have to be persisted for 4–nine months in sufferers with a primary episode of essential despair that turned into now no longer related to tremendous suicidality or catastrophic outcomes. In the ones who've had 2 or extra episodes of despair, an extended direction of upkeep remedy can also additionally show beneficial.

In 2011, the American Psychiatric Association (APA) up to date its Practice Guideline for the Treatment of Patients with Major Depressive Disorder. The 2011 APA guiding principle emphasizes the want to customize a remedy plan for every affected person primarily based totally on a cautious evaluation of signs, along with score scale measurements administered via way of means of a clinician or the affected person, in addition to an evaluation of healing advantages and facet consequences.

Treatment have to maximize affected person feature inside unique and practical goals. The preliminary modality has to be selected on the premise of the following:

Manufactured by Amazon.ca
Bolton, ON

30982090R00103